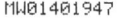

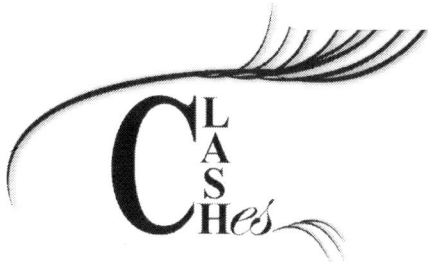

The Black & White Lash Manual
Clashes Eyelash Extension Artist Training Manual 2nd Edition

In black & white to save you money, this is your complete guide to the anatomy and physiology of the eye and natural eyelashes, proper professional eyelash extension products, extension application methods, including Russian Volume fan building instructions, and everything else you need to know in order to become an eyelash extension artist!

Authored by Chrystal Ladouceur
Illustrations by Dani Teitsma

Copyright © 2017 Chrystal Ladouceur
All rights reserved.
ISBN-10: 1974023273
ISBN-13: 978-1974023271
Illustrations by Dani Tietsma
Edited by Sheilah Egan

Previous Edition Information
Eyelash Extension Artist Training Manual
Published February 7 2017
ISBN-10: 1542929407
ISBN-13: 978-1542929400
Illustrations by Dani Tietsma
Edited by Sheilah Egan

For Bailey – because you can grow up to be anything you want to be and to do anything you want to do.

Contents

Contents	5
1. Introduction	11
2. Anatomy of the Eyeball	13
The Cornea	13
The Sclera	14
The Conjunctiva	14
The Iris & Pupil	14
The Lens	14
The Retina	15
The Macula & Fovea Centralis	15
The Optic Nerve	15
The Vitreous Body	15
How the Eye Works	15
Chapter Summary Points	16
Definitions	16
3. Anatomy & Physiology of the Eyelashes	17
Structure of an Eyelash	17
Meibomian Glands & Meibum	18
Eyelash Growth Cycle	19
Seasonal Shedding	20
Chapter Summary Points	20
Definitions	21
4. Diseases & Disorders Involving the Eyes & Eyelashes	22
Conjunctivitis	22
Dry Eye Syndrome	23
Stys & Chalazia	24
Xanthelasma & Milia	24
Cataract	25
Glaucoma	25
Diabetic Retinopathy	26
Madarosis	26
Trichotillomania	27
Traction Alopecia	27
Blepharitis	27
Distichiasis & Trichiasis	28
Crab Lice Infestation	28
Demodex Folliculorum	29
Chapter Summary Points	29
Definitions	29
5. Contraindications to Eyelash Extensions	30
Absolute Contraindications	30
Subjective Contraindications	31
Informed Consent	32

The Patch or Spot Test	33
Allergies	33
Managing Allergic Reactions	34
Chapter Summary Points	35
Definitions	36

6. Ministry of Health Disease Control in B.C. — 37

General Operation Guidelines	37
Administering Drugs or Eye Drops	38
Equipment	39
Infection Control	39
Sterilization & Disinfection	40
High-Level Disinfection	40
High-Level Disinfection with Bleach	41
Other Materials	41
Personnel	41
Chapter Summary Points	42
Definitions	42

7. Safety & First Aid — 43

General Product Precautions	43
Cyanoacrylate Cautions	44
First Aid for Product Eye Contact	45
First Aid for Product Skin Contact	45
First Aid for Product Inhalation	45
First Aid for Product Ingestion	46
Chapter Summary Points	46
Definitions	47

8. Professional Eyelash Extension Products — 48

Tweezers	48
Fans & Puffers	49
Glue Carriers	49
Lash Rings or Bulbs	49
Under Eyelid Lash Barriers	50
Cosmetic Scissors	50
Disposable Eyelash Wands	51
Micro Brushes	51
Cotton Swabs	52
Eyelash Extensions	52
Eyelash Cleansers & Primers	55
Eyelash Extension Glue	56
Eyelash Adhesive Removers	58
Nano Misters	59
Thermometers & Hygrometers	59
Chapter Summary Points	59
Definitions	60

9. Client Consultation & Consent — 61

Client Considerations	62
Client's Daily Activity & After Care	62
Cleansing & Brushing Lash Extensions	63
Mild Eyelash Cleanser	64
Chapter Summary Points	64
Definitions	64

10. Station Set Up — 65

Lashing Environment Temperature & Humidity	65
Client Comfort	65
Artist's Comfort	66
Tools & Supplies	67
Chapter Summary Points	68
Definitions	68

11. Eyelash Extension Application — 69

Selecting Safe Extension Lengths, Widths & Weights	69
Classic Lash Selection	71
Lash Mapping	72
Popular Eyelash Extension Maps	74
Natural Eye Shapes & Choosing Lash Styles	75
Round, Oval or Almond Shaped Eyes	76
Close Set Eyes	76
Wide Set Eyes	76
Hooded Eyes	77
Monolid	77
Deep Set Eyes	78
Down Turned Eyes	78
Apply Lower Lash Barrier	78
Cleanse & Prime Natural Lashes	81
Determine Application Pattern & Isolate Natural Eyelash	82
Apply Extensions	83
Inspection & Lash Separation	85
Final Comb Through, Setting & Finishing Up	86
Classic Extension Application Step-by-Step	87
Fill Appointment Applications	87
Fill Appointment Step-by-Step	88
Application Tips & Tricks	89
Hooded Eyelids & Lash Angles	89
Taping Up	90
Increasing Glue Longevity	90
Glue Holder Clean Up	91
Mid-Application Breaks	92
Chapter Summary Points	92
Definitions	92

12. Volume & Russian Volume Application — 93

Understanding Volume Weight	95
Understanding Russian Volume Fan Bonding	97

Building Volume Fans	97
Building Volume Fans Method 1	98
Building Volume Fans Method 2	98
Building Volume Fans Method 3	98
Building Volume Fans Method 4	99
Building Volume Fans Method 5	99
Practicing Russian Volume	100
Chapter Summary Points	101
Definitions	101

13. Eyelash Extension Removal — 102

Individual Extension Removal	102
Complete Extension Removal	104
Complete Extension Removal Step-by-Step	105
Self Removal of Eyelashes	106
Chapter Summary Points	107

14. Whoops! Fixing Things that have Gone Wrong — 108

Under Eye Pad Won't Stick	108
Lashes Stick Together During Application	108
Lashes Keep Sticking to the Under Eye Pad	109
Lashes or Glue Gets Stuck To Upper Eyelid	110
Old Extension Twists and/or Weighs the Lash Down	111
Client Feels the Product is in Their Eye	111
There is a Gap in the Natural Lashes	112
Clients Eyes Are Twitchy While you Work	113
Client Can't Open Eye as a Top Lash Stuck to the Bottom	114
Eyelash Extensions Fall Out Prematurely	114
Eyelash Extensions Lose their Curl	116
Eyelash Extensions are Itchy or Uncomfortable	116
Generalized Red Eyes (Conjunctivitis) After Eyelash Extensions Applied	117
Localized Red Eyes (Conjunctivitis) / Bruised Eyeball	117
Chapter Summary Points	118
Definitions	119

15. Bad Eyelash Extensions / Good Eyelash Extensions — 120

16. Closing Notes — 123

Appendix — 125

Intake Form	126
Liability Waiver	129
Client Record – Lash History	133
After Care Check List	134

References & Further Learning Materials — 135

1. Introduction

Congratulations on your choice to become an eyelash extension artist! This is the most comprehensive training manual on professional eyelash extensions available. With the purchase of this book, you are well on your way to becoming an expert in the field. This book was created with in-depth information on the anatomy of the eye, one of the human body's most important organs, a close look at the human eyelash growth cycles, vital information for any eyelash extension artist to have, and eye diseases or conditions that may make a person a poor candidate for eyelash extension applications. This is to ensure that you are keeping your client's best interests in mind throughout your career as an eyelash extension artist. This book also covers professional materials and supplies available, the application process itself, the proper removal of eyelash extensions and other detailed information that you should have as an eyelash extension artist. While the government guidelines and regulations discussed in this book originate from the government of British Columbia, Canada, the lessons learned and the practices encouraged can be used anywhere in the world – so long as you're also abiding by your own government regulations!

I've created this book because the eyelash extension industry is not currently regulated in Canada. There are no standards of practice, and no consumer guarantees. Educational resources are sparse and vary dramatically in quality. Applying eyelash extensions requires that adhesives similar to Krazy Glue are used just millimeters from the eye of your client. And because the industry is not regulated, anyone can offer eyelash extension services, whether or not they are properly trained to do so! As a result, the potential for things to go wrong are vast and wide. Adverse affects can be cosmetic, caused by poor application technique or style choice. They can be complicated, such as complete loss of natural eyelashes, leaving the surface of the eye vulnerable to foreign bodies such as microbes and dust. Or they can be severe such as serious allergic reactions that require immediate medical attention. Without regulation, there are no guarantees that protect the public or the eyelash extension artist from any potential adverse effects. What we can do as personal service providers is be aware of the potential for things to go wrong. We can have knowledge of what those things are so that we can actively try to prevent them from happening, and if they do happen, we can know how to administer first aid. Finally, what we must do is share that knowledge with our clients so they are informed before we begin the application process.

The more information you have, the more prepared and confident you will be in using your new skills. This comprehensive manual will provide you with all of the information you need in order to start practicing the hands-on application of semi-permanent eyelash extensions. Read this book through from beginning to end and then keep it on hand as a reference guide in case you forget a step in the future. In the back of this book, you'll find form templates you may copy and modify for your personal use as you get started working on real clients.

However detailed as this book is, you cannot become an expert in the eyelash extension application process without proper hands-on practice. Reading this book in its entirety certainly does not replace a hands-on in-person course. I recommend reviewing this book as foundational information prior to, or as companion piece, to your hands-on training, and not as a replacement for it!

2. Anatomy of the Eyeball

The eyeball is your organ of sight. It sits within the bony cavity of the skull known as the orbit, where it is moved by ocular muscles and is protected by accessory structures including muscles, fascia, eyebrows, eyelashes, eyelids, and the lacrimal apparatus. The eye has a number of components, which include (but are not limited to) the cornea, the sclera, the conjunctiva, the iris, the lens and pupil, the retina, macula and fovea centralis, the optic nerve, and the vitreous body. Lets take a look at each of these parts:

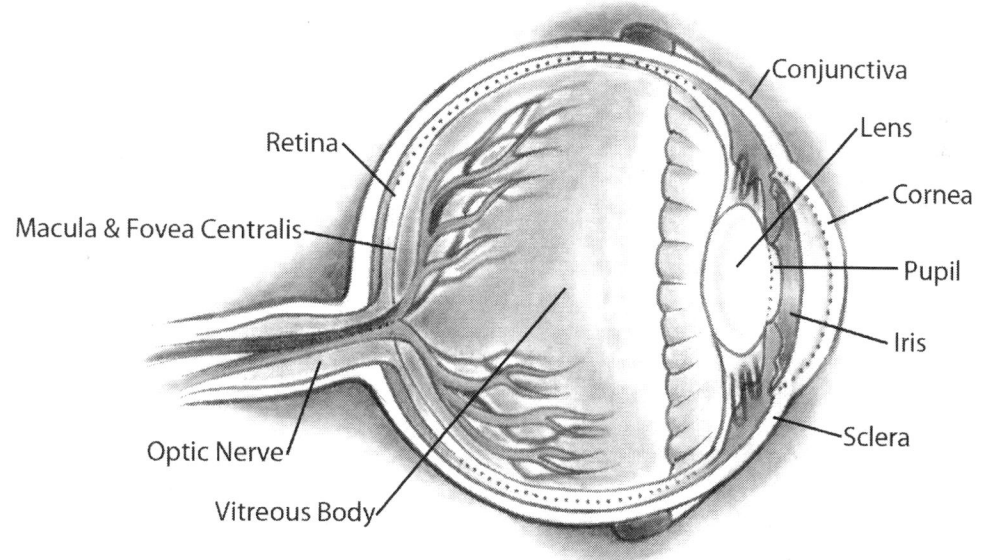

The Cornea

The cornea is the clear front window of the eye that transmits and focuses light into the eye. It covers the iris, pupil and the anterior chamber of the eye, which aids it in transmitting and focusing light. While the cornea is a fixed structure, it contributes most to the eye's focusing power. Lasik, the popular laser surgery to correct nearsightedness, farsightedness and/or astigmatism, focuses on reshaping the cornea.

The Sclera

The sclera is the outer white layer of the eye and as such it's often referred to as simply the white of the eye. It is an opaque, fibrous, protective layer of the eye containing collagen and elastic fiber. At the front of the eye, it is continuous with the cornea.

The Conjunctiva

The conjunctiva is the mucus membrane that covers the sclera and lines the inside of the eyelid. It helps lubricate the eye by producing mucus and tears. It is believed to contribute to immune surveillance, the patrolling of the body to recognize and destroy invading pathogens or damaged cells. It also helps prevent microbes from entering the eye. The conjunctiva is highly vascularized, which means it has a lot of blood vessels. When someone's eyes look bloodshot, it is the conjunctiva that creates the reddened appearance.

The Iris & Pupil

The iris is the thin, circular, colored structure in the eye that is responsible for controlling the diameter of the pupil. The pupil is the dark aperture (or hole) in the center of the iris. By changing the size of the pupil, the iris helps regulate the amount of light that enters the eye and reaches the retina. The iris is usually strongly pigmented with color, defining the color of the eye usually as brown, hazel, green, grey or blue. A lack of pigmentation in the iris results in the pinkish-white colored eye seen in albinism.

The Lens

The lens is a transparent, biconvex (or football-shaped) structure inside the eye that along with the cornea, focuses light rays onto the retina. The lens changes shape to alter the focal distance of the eye so that it can focus on objects at various distances. This works in a way that resembles focusing a photographic camera in order to take a picture. A clouding of the lens of the eye, most commonly occurring due to aging, is known as a cataract.

The Retina
The retina is a complex structure of light-sensitive tissue. It contains two types of photosensitive cells: rods and cones. The retina also consists of a thin layer of nerves that line the back of the eye. Light striking the retina triggers nerve impulses that are sent to various visual centers of the brain through the fibers of the optic nerve. An image is produced by patterned electrical impulses created by the retina, which are then processed by the neuronal system and the brain to form vision.

The Macula & Fovea Centralis
The macula is a small central area of the retina that contains special light-sensitive cells. Near the center of the macula is the fovea centralis, a small pit that contains a concentration of cone cells. This specific area is responsible for the high-resolution, color vision that is possible in good light.

The Optic Nerve
The optic nerve connects the eye to the brain. It transmits visual information formed by the retina to the visual cortex of the brain, where your brain constructs the images you see.

The Vitreous Body
The vitreous body is the clear, jelly-like substance that fills the space between the lens of the eye and the retina. This transparent, colorless, gelatinous mass is present at birth. Unlike other fluids of the body and eye, which are continuously replenished, the vitreous body is stagnant and unchanging throughout life. Floaters are small spots that drift through the field of vision sometimes casting shadows. These tend to appear as we age and are caused by tiny flecks of the protein collagen floating loose in the vitreous body.

How the Eye Works
The human eye works a lot like a digital camera. Light is focused by the cornea and lens, which together work much like that of a camera lens. The iris functions like the diaphragm of a camera, adjusting the size of the

pupil to control the amount of light that reaches the retina on the back of the eye. The retina acts like the image sensor of a digital camera, converting optical images into electric impulses that are then interpreted by the visual cortex of the brain.

Chapter Summary Points
- The eyeball is one of your most vital organs, responsible for sight.
- The eyeball is a complex organ that is made of many different structures.
- The eyeball is protected by a number of other accessory structures including the eyelashes.
- The superficial structures of the eyeball include the sclera and cornea, and are covered by the conjunctiva.

Definitions

Ocular	of or connected with the eyes or vision
Fascia	connective tissue beneath the skin that attaches, stabilizes, encloses and separates muscles and other internal organs
Lacrimal apparatus	the system responsible for tear production and drainage
Pathogens	a bacterium, virus, or other microorganism that can cause disease
Vascularized	provide (a tissue or structure) with vessels, especially blood vessels; make vascular
Pigmented	color (something) with or as if with pigment

3. Anatomy & Physiology of the Eyelashes

Some of the more feminine features of the face, and the most important structures for an eyelash extension artist, are the eyelashes, often simply referred to as lashes. An eyelash is one of the hairs that grow at the edge of the eyelids. They serve to protect the eye from debris and are sensitive to touch. They provide a warning when an object is near to the eye, and in response to that warning, the eyelids close by reflex.

If the eyelashes are pulled out, they can take up to eight weeks to grow back. Constant pulling may damage the growing mechanism and lead to permanent damage or complete eyelash loss, known as Madarosis. Madarosis is one of the disorders involving the eyelashes that we will look at in the next chapter. For now, let's take a closer look at the anatomy and physiology of the eyelash.

Structure of an Eyelash

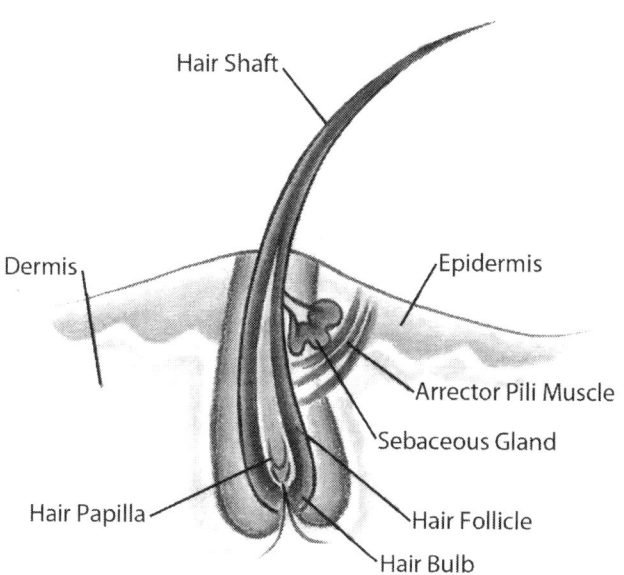

Composed of proteins such as melanin and keratin, and a small amount of water, each eyelash consists of multiple parts. The parts of the eyelash include the hair shaft, which is the long body of the lash that you can see above the epidermis, or skin. This is the part of the eyelash that an eyelash extension is adhered to. Each eyelash, like all of your body hair, has it's own arrector pili muscle. This is the tiny muscle that is responsible for your hairs standing on edge when you get the shivers! Also connected to each of the eyelashes are two glands, the sebaceous gland and the sudiferous gland. The sebaceous gland secretes lubricating oil known as sebum, while the sudiferous gland produces sweat. The hair follicle is a sheath of cells and connective tissue that surrounds the root of the hair. The bulb is the area from which the hair begins to grow. The bulb is shaped around the papilla, the knob-like indentation on the bottom of the bulb. The papilla contains vascular loops, or blood vessels, that provide nourishment to the hair.

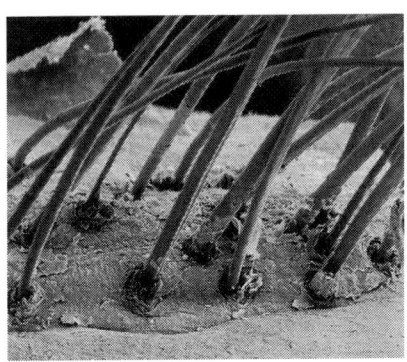

Under a microscope we can see that at the edge of the eyelids, eyelashes grow in approximately three rows. The upper lid has on average 70 to 150 lashes, while the lower lid has between 60 and 80 lashes. The upper lashes curve upwards while the lower lashes curve down. This helps protect the eye from dust and other foreign particles.

Meibomian Glands & Meibum

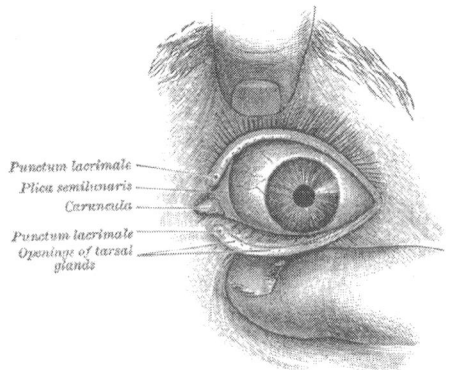

Between the lash line and the eyeball is the rim of the eyelid. The rim of the eyelid is composed of Meibomian glands, referred to in the above

- We lose more eyelashes in the spring and summer than in the winter or autumn months.

Definitions

Melanin	dark brown to black pigment occurring in the hair, skin and iris of the eye
Keratin	fibrous protein forming the main structural constituent of hair and nails
Epidermis	surface layer of the skin that overlays the dermis
Anagen	active growth phase of hair follicles
Catagen	transitional phase of the hair growth cycle when the follicle is shrinking
Telogen	resting phase of the hair growth cycle

4. Diseases & Disorders Involving the Eyes & Eyelashes

There are multiple diseases and disorders involving the eyes and eyelashes that an eyelash extension artist should be aware of. While some of these conditions are more common than others, you may come across any of these at any given time. Some of them are contraindications for eyelash extensions. We will look closely at specific contraindications in the next chapter. For now, lets take a look at some of these diseases and disorders.

Conjunctivitis

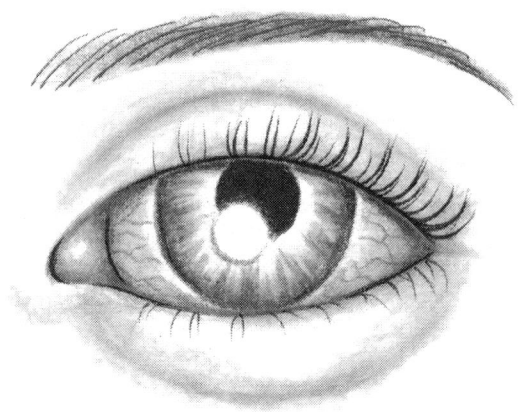

Conjunctivitis translates to inflammation of the conjunctiva. It is often simply referred to as pinkeye because, as suggested, it makes the white of the eye appear to be the color pink. There are a number of different potential causes of conjunctivitis, including viruses, bacteria, allergies or irritants. Because it's impossible for us to know what the cause of someone's pinkeye actually is without a doctor's diagnoses, you should not apply eyelash extensions to someone who is actively presenting with it. The person suffering this may be contagious, and the application procedure, and any of the supplies used, may irritate it further and make the clients eyes worse. If a client arrives for their appointment with pinkeye, ask them to postpone their appointment until the eyes have cleared up and are in good health again.

It is important to note here that temporary conjunctivitis is a normal response for some people with sensitive eyes, to having eyelash extensions applied. We will discuss this in more detail later in the book.

Dry Eye Syndrome

Dry eye syndrome, technically referred to as keratoconjunctivitis sicca, or just KCS, is a condition of having dry eyes. It's sometimes paired with discharge or frequent tearing. While tearing may seem like a paradox to dry eyes, it is the body's natural response to sensing a dry mucous layer on the eye. In an effort to correct the dry mucous layer, the body will create tears. Dry eye syndrome may also simply be caused by an inability to produce a sufficient amount of tears in the first place, or tears that evaporate much too quickly. Regardless of the cause, symptoms include burning and stinging sensations, along with redness of the eye. Sufferers may also have easily fatigued eyes and blurred vision.

While dry eye syndrome is common, affecting between 5%-34% of the population, the symptoms can range from mild and occasional to severe and continuous. Many people who suffer this condition opt not to wear makeup because of either frequent tearing, or the frequent need for artificial tears or eye drops in order to sooth the dry eyes. Because makeup runs, sufferers of dry eye syndrome may be perfect candidates for eyelash extensions, as once applied no make-up is needed to give the lashes a full, fully made-up look. At the same time, the frequent tearing or use of artificial tears may lead to premature breakdown of the adhesives used, so the client may find the lashes do not last as long as they otherwise would. If the eyes are tearing during the application process, the bond between the natural hair and the eyelash extension may be weak to begin with.

Another consideration for the client who suffers dry eyes is the necessity not to irritate an already irritated eye. Prior to the application, the client must be advised of possible irritation due to adhesives and other chemicals used. Those who suffer dry eyes are prime candidates for pre-application spot tests. We will cover informed client consent and spot tests in a later chapter.

Stys & Chalazia

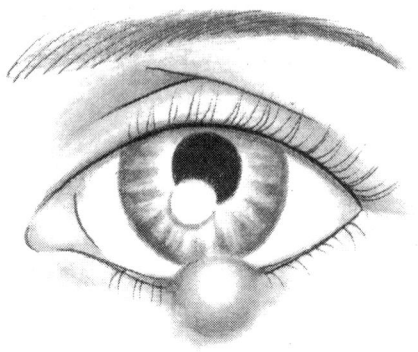
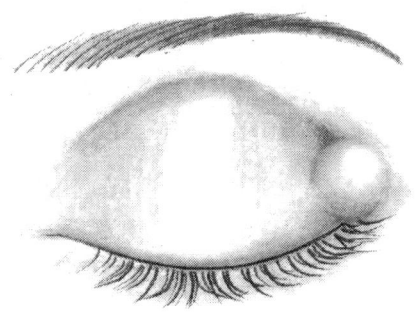

Stys and chalazia are infected sweat or oil glands on either the lower or upper eyelid; both conditions present as red, swollen bumps on the eyelids. A sty is caused by a staphylococcus aureus (or just staph for short) bacterial infection. Chalazia are blocked oil glands of the eyelid. The staphylococcus aureus bacteria is highly contagious and without a doctor's diagnoses, you have no way of knowing if it is, or is not, the cause of this condition. As such, without a doctor's consent you should not be applying eyelash extensions to someone who appears to have either of these until the condition has cleared up and there are no longer any signs of infection or irritation.

Xanthelasma & Milia

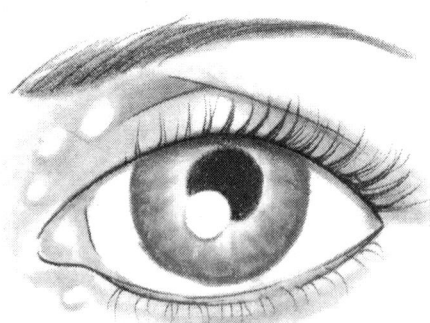
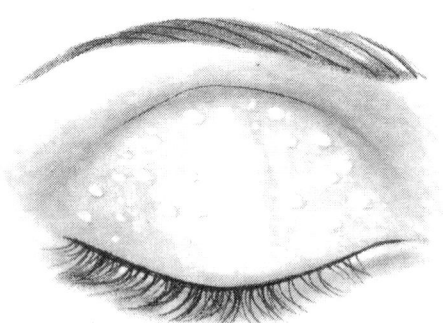

Xanthelasma, as shown in the illustration on the left, is a yellowish deposit of fat underneath the skin usually on, or around, the eyelids. It is often seen in people with high cholesterol levels, but also may simply have ethnic origins. Xanthelasma are not painful or harmful and can be removed by a doctor for cosmetic reasons, if necessary.

Milia, shown in the previous drawing on the right, are often referred to as milk spots. Milia occur when skin cells don't slough off normally and become trapped at the base of the sweat glands. This is often seen in infants but can also present in adults. It results in tiny white cysts on the upper eyelid. While in children Milia tend to disappear in a few weeks on their own, adults may need to seek the care of a physician to have them removed. They are not harmful or contagious.

Cataract

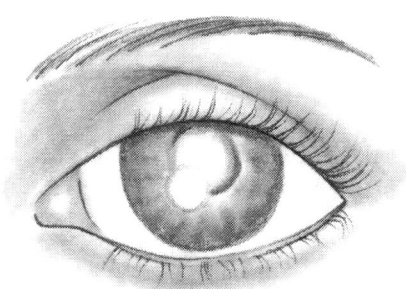

Cataract is the clouding of the eye's natural lens. This is the most common cause of vision loss in people over the age of 40 and is the principal cause of blindness worldwide. Cataract is not harmful or contagious.

Glaucoma

Glaucoma referrers to a group of related eye disorders that all cause damage to the optic nerve. As previously discussed, this is the nerve that carries information from the eye to the brain. In most cases, glaucoma is usually associated with higher than normal pressure inside the eye, a condition called ocular hypertension. It can also occur with normal pressure inside the eye. Glaucoma is the second-leading cause of blindness in the U.S.

The drug Bimatoprost is a prostaglandin analog drug designed to treat glaucoma by reducing intraocular pressure. Throughout testing and research studies, it was discovered to increase eyelash diameter, density and length leading to an increase in overall eyelash growth, by way of extending the telogen phase of the lash growth cycle. Since, eyelash growth serums have been developed using similar formulas. The most common prescription drug used for eyelash growth is branded as Latisse.

Diabetic Retinopathy

Diabetic Retinopathy is vision-threatening damage to the retina of the eye that is caused by diabetes. While many cases could be prevented with regular eye exams and appropriate treatment, it is still one of the leading causes of blindness among working-age Americans.

Madarosis

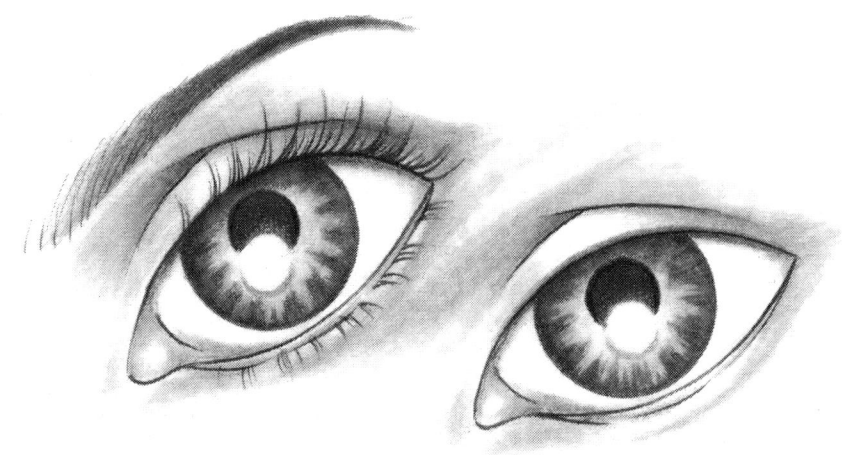

Madarosis is the loss of the eyelashes and sometimes the eyebrows. It may be caused by various things, including dermatologic conditions like late stage alopecia (baldness), nutritional defects, infections, trauma as in the frequent pulling out of eyelashes, genetics, autoimmune disorders and perhaps most commonly, as a side effect to certain medications. This is often observed in cancer patients who are undergoing chemotherapy. People suffering from Madarosis cannot have eyelash extension applied. Professional eyelash extensions must be applied to the natural eyelash and cannot be applied to the skin of the eyelid.

Trichotillomania

Trichotillomania, also called hair-pulling disorder, is a compulsive desire to pull one's own hair out. This is a psychological disorder that involves recurrent, irresistible urges to pull out from the scalp, eyebrows, eyelashes or other areas of the body. Often, the person suffering this condition has a strong desire to stop. They may be ashamed of their condition, leading them to deny it or to refrain from disclosing it.

People with Trichotillomania may be prime candidates for eyelash extensions; however, as the extensions fall out, or if they are uncomfortable in any way, their desire to pull out the remaining lashes may be increased. For some, keeping their extensions full with regular fill appointments is enough to prevent them from pulling. For others, the compulsion is just too strong so they become contraindicated to the service.

Traction Alopecia

Traction alopecia is the term given to the loss of hair due to it being pulled out. Eyelash extension artists will often see this in clients who have had lash extension done by non-skilled technicians without care. This condition is avoided through proper eyelash isolation and lash application, as we will discuss later.

Blepharitis

Blepharitis is a common eye condition that presents as inflammation of the eyelids, most often right where the eyelashes grow. A number of diseases and conditions can lead to Blepharitis, including blocked oil glands at the bases of the eyelashes, bacterial infections and allergies. Blepharitis can be caused by an eyelash extension client's poor hygiene. They may think they are protecting their eyelash extensions by not washing them, but instead they are creating a perfect environment for bacteria to grow between the eyelid and the eyelash extension's adhesive bond. It's important to advise your clients to wash their eyelashes.

The severity of Blepharitis can vary from case-to-case and depending on the cause. Blepharitis almost always results in irritated, itchy, reddened eyelids. Similar to Conjunctivitis, Blepharitis can be highly contagious and easily irritated further; as such, you should not apply eyelash extensions to someone who is suffering this condition and you should remove eyelash extensions from someone who develops blepharitis after the extensions have been applied.

Distichiasis & Trichiasis

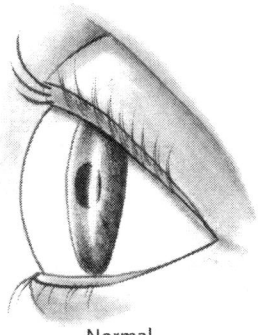
Normal

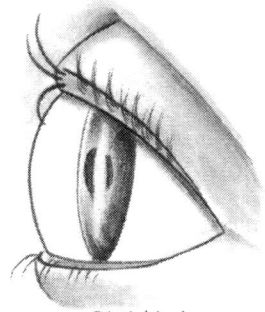
Distichiasis

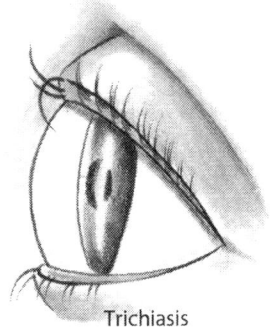
Trichiasis

Distichiasis is condition in which an extra row of eyelashes emerges. The lashes can be fine and well tolerated or coarser and a threat to the cornea. Trichiasis is a condition in which the eyelashes emerging from their normal origin curve inward towards the cornea. The cause of Trichiasis is sometimes unknown, but it can also be the result of chronic inflammatory conditions.

Crab Lice Infestation

A crab louse is a parasitic insect that feeds exclusively on blood. Crab lice (louse is singular) infestations are often found in pubic hair, however, they can also be found in the eyelashes and eyebrows. The main symptom sufferers' present with is itching and irritation of the eyes and eyelashes. These symptoms cause the infected person to rub or scratch the eyes. Crab lice infections are highly contagious and you should not be applying eyelash extensions to someone who is suffering this condition. If you suspect a client has this condition, suggest they see a medical doctor.

Demodex Folliculorum

Demodex Folliculorum is a species of face mite. These mites are normally found in human hair follicles, especially around the eyelashes and eyebrows. These mites are also found on dogs. They vary in size from 0.1mm to 0.4mm long and are semi-transparent so you cannot see them with the naked eye. They are not harmful; however, outbreaks caused by a weakened immune system or stress, can lead to harm, including the condition mange that is seen in dogs.

Chapter Summary Points

- There are plenty of diseases and conditions that affect the eyes and eyelashes.
- Some conditions are contraindicated to the eyelash extension procedure.
- Some conditions create prime candidates for eyelash extensions, with careful considerations.
- An eyelash extension artist should be familiar with eye conditions and diseases.

Definitions

Contraindication	a condition or factor that serves as a reason to withhold a treatment due to the harm that it would cause the patient
-itis	a medical suffix that means "inflammation of"
Dermatologic	the branch of medicine dealing with the skin, nails, hair and its diseases
Alopecia	the partial or complete absence of hair from areas of the body where it normally grows; baldness
Parasite	an organism that lives in or on another organism (its host) and benefits by deriving nutrients at the host's expense

5. Contraindications to Eyelash Extensions

There are some very specific absolute contraindications to eyelash extension application. There are also situations where you need to use your best judgment to decide whether or not the service is suited for your client, and if you can proceed to apply eyelash extensions with or without modifications. Absolute contraindications include any reasons why applying professional eyelash extensions may cause harm to your client, your future clients, or yourself. Subjective contraindications include any situations where the potential benefits outweigh the potential consequences. You must only proceed to apply eyelash extensions with the informed consent of your client.

Absolute Contraindications

If your client is suffering any eye disease or condition that may be contagious, you cannot apply eyelash extensions. By proceeding with the application, you would be putting yourself and your future clients at risk, regardless of how thorough your sterilization procedures are.

Any eye condition that presents as a red, swollen, or inflamed condition has the potential to be further irritated by the application process, or any of the products used, is absolutely contraindicated. You should not attempt to apply eyelash extensions to any client who has obvious signs of infection or irritation. These signs include redness of the eyes and/or eyelids, puffiness around the eyes, and/or severe itching of the eyes or eyelids.

Also absolutely contraindicated to professional eyelash extensions are clients who for whatever reason suffer madarosis, or a lack of eyelashes. Professional eyelash extensions must be applied to a natural eyelash. The skin of the eyelid is not suitable for the semi-permanent bonding adhesives used. The glues used can damage the skin itself, and lead to other severe adverse reactions. Also, because of the complex oil secreting, sweating nature of skin, any bond applied would not last. Consider a time in your life when you may have accidently applied Krazy glue, or some permanent pigment like ink or paint, to your hand or somewhere else on your body directly to the skin. Even without washing, in a matter of days or hours, it's gone. The skin secretes oils and sweat, which leads to shedding of whatever substance was applied to its surface.

Absolutely contraindicated conditions include conjunctivitis (pinkeye), stys, chalazia, and any other red, swollen bumps of the eyelids, madarosis, blepharitis and crab lice infestations. Anything that results in red, puffy or severely itchy eyes, or that clearly looks like an infection, should be avoided.

Subjective Contraindications

Situations where the benefits of having eyelash extensions applied outweigh any potential consequences require your careful consideration, and the detailed, informed consent of your client prior to the application process. This includes people who have possible or known sensitivities to any of the products used; people who are recovering from madarosis; people who regularly use eye drops or false tears; and people who have lifestyles that may result in the premature breakdown of the adhesives used.

The eyelash application procedure requires the use of a number of products with chemical components that we will discuss later. Many people are sensitive to these types of products, and because they are being used in close proximity to the eye, a very sensitive organ, even those who don't normally suffer reactions may find some temporary discomfort during, or immediately after, the application process. Mild reactions may present as a temporary conjunctivitis that lasts a few minutes to a few hours, or even days. Severe reactions may result in extreme discomfort, swelling of the eyelids and require immediate removal of the eyelashes as well as medical attention. All clients must be informed of the potential for adverse reactions. Clients with known sensitivities, or who may suffer adverse reactions, should have a patch test done prior to the full application process.

Special consideration should also be given to clients who have undergone chemotherapy, or present with any other condition that caused hair loss and are recovering from madarosis at the time of their eyelash extension appointment. Eyelash extensions may serve to increase self-confidence and encourage a sense of normalcy, which can increase the quality of life and reduce some stress for a cancer survivor. As awesome as it is that an eyelash extension artist can help in such a way, it is important to recall that each professional eyelash extension must be applied to a natural lash and cannot be applied to skin, so some natural eyelashes must exist before you can proceed with application.

Finally, some people live lives that simply make them poor candidates for professional eyelash extensions. People who are regular swimmers, or who spend large portions of their lives in high humidity or high heat atmospheres like steam rooms or saunas, or people who regularly use false tears or eye drops, such as those who suffer dry eye syndrome, must be made aware that lash retention is reduced in these situations. Adhesives are broken down more quickly when in constant contact with water, saline solutions, and high temperatures. High temperatures may deform the extensions themselves, often reducing the curl, and extremely high temperatures will melt or burn the eyelash extensions and the natural lashes. The other lifestyle conditions may simply result in a more frequent need for fill appointments.

Informed Consent

Within the health industry, the number one contraindication is not having proper informed consent from a patient. In British Columbia, this applies to the aesthetic industry as well. You simply cannot do a procedure, or proceed with a personal service, without proper informed consent from your client. This means that your client should be aware of, and should fully understand, exactly what you intend to do. They must be aware of all possible outcomes, good and bad, as well as any corrective procedures in place.

As the service provider, it is your responsibility to give the client as much information as possible and to allow them to make the decision to proceed with the service you are offering. Failing to properly obtain informed consent from a client may lead to serious legal ramifications for you in the event that something should go wrong. For this reason, you should obtain informed consent both verbally, through discussion with your client, and in writing, in the form of a signed liability waiver. There is a sample simple liability waiver in the appendix of this book that you may modify to your needs and use. However, it is in your best interest to seek legal consultation to make sure the waiver is applicable to your situation. You may also consider contacting your local insurance broker in order to protect yourself against any potential damages awarded to a client in case of negligence.

The Patch or Spot Test

In order to minimize or prevent serious adverse reactions, you should always offer to perform a patch test at least 24 to 48 hours before the full application of eyelash extensions, especially for clients with known sensitivities, new clients, or if you change any of the products that you use.

A patch test follows the exact eyelash extension application procedure, using all of the same equipment and products that you would use during a regular application. This includes taping off the bottom lashes, cleansing and priming of the upper lashes, and then the actual application of just 2 to 3 individual lashes at the outside of the eye(s). The client is then asked to be mindful of any adverse reactions over the next few days. In the event of any adverse reactions, the test lashes should be removed and you should not go forward with the full application. If no adverse reaction is noted, proceed to book the regular application appointment.

The patch test should take less than 20 minutes to complete. It is not recommended that you charge for this service as doing a patch test is in both your and your client's best interest. It may save you time and money in the future.

Allergies

An allergic reaction is hypersensitivity so a substance that comes into contact with the body. Any substance that causes an allergic reaction is called an allergen. In the eyelash extension industry, people will sometimes react to the adhesives, the extensions or the other products that we use. While many allergic reactions may start out mild, repeat exposure to an allergen causes a graded response in the body, that gets worse with each instance of exposure, which can eventually lead to the most severe form of an allergy, anaphylaxis (or anaphylactic shock). Anaphylaxis is a medical emergency. In less than 15 minutes it can cause death.

People with known allergies carry an EpiPen in case of accidental contact with an allergen. They know to contact emergency medical services immediately should they ever need to use the EpiPen, as the EpiPen's effects are temporary. Most severe allergic reactions will occur within seconds or minutes after exposure to the allergen, but reactions may less commonly happen hours, or days even, after contact.

In the eyelash extension industry, some clients will develop allergies only after the repeat exposure of wearing eyelash extensions for years. And since the products used in eyelash extensions are new or novel to many other people, it can sometimes take a few days for a notable reaction to occur, even the first time. A patch test done a few days prior to the extension application does not guarantee that no reaction will ever occur. It simply adds a cushion of confidence that you may apply a set of eyelash extensions on the client without an immediate concern for a full-blown emergency reaction.

Managing Allergic Reactions

Allergic reactions are said to happen in up to 5% of all eyelash extension applications. This is about 1 for every 20 clients. They are most common in people who have never had eyelash extensions applied, but they can develop in anyone, even people who have been having eyelash extension applied for years.

Allergic reactions to eyelash extensions present as red, extremely puffy, swollen upper and lower, eyelids. The reaction may start to occur while you are still applying the extensions or it may occur hours or even days later. The reaction may initially start only in one eye. In most cases, the reaction is sooner than later, but sometimes the client will wait until eyes are almost swollen shut before they start to consider removal.

Doctors may refuse to treat people until the eyelash extensions are removed. While this may seem rather harsh at first, it makes sense, as the extensions are the allergen so until they are removed, any treatment would be pointless. It is extremely important for this reason that you always make yourself available to do an emergency eyelash removal, especially in the hours immediately after applying a new set for the very first time on someone.

Patch tests are designed to help reduce the number of full-blown allergic reactions you may encounter. Always do a patch test on a new client. If an allergic reaction occurs, have your client consult with a pharmacist or a nurse about taking an over the counter antihistamine like Benyadryl. You cannot recommend the client take any medication, as you are not a registered health professional. We will discuss this in a later chapter. For now, know you can suggest that the client speak to a health professional regarding antihistamines and you should do so in the event of an allergic reaction. Then immediately follow the steps for extension removal and have your client seek medical care. You should never attempt to re-apply the extensions on someone who has had an allergic response. Allergic responses are graded and get worse with every instance of contact with the allergen. On my website, as linked in the resource section of this book, there is a detailed explanation of how and why allergic reactions occur.

In British Columbia, the telephone number to the nurse's hotline is 811. You should keep this number handy and give it to your clients if necessary.

Chapter Summary Points

- Absolute contraindications include any reasons why the application may cause harm to your client, your future clients, or yourself.
- Subjective contraindications include any situations where the potential benefits outweigh the potential consequences.
- You cannot proceed with a personal service without proper informed consent from your client.
- A patch test should be offered to new clients and to all clients any time you change products.

- People will sometimes react to the adhesives, the extensions or the other products that we use.
- A patch test done a few days prior to the extension application does not guarantee that no reaction will ever occur.
- Allergies can happen to any client, even those who have had eyelash extensions for years.
- In British Columbia, the telephone number to the nurse's hotline is 811.

Definitions

Absolute contraindication	offering this service may cause harm to your client, your future client or yourself. Do not apply eyelash extensions
Subjective contraindication	offering this service may be possible with modification and caution
Informed consent	permission granted in the knowledge of the possible consequences, typically that which is given by a client to a personal service provider for service with full knowledge of the possible risks and benefits
Liability waiver	a legal document that a person who participates in an activity may sign to acknowledge the risks involved in his or her participation
Allergen	a substance that causes an allergic reaction
Anaphylaxis	a severe, potentially life-threatening allergic reaction
EpiPen	a brand name for an epinephrine auto-injector device used to manage potentially life-threatening anaphylactic reactions to allergens

6. Ministry of Health Disease Control in B.C.

Our government considers eyelash extension application as a personal service. As such, the place in which you are offering this service is considered a Personal Service Establishment (PSE) and it must comply with Canada Health Act's Personal Service Establishments Regulation. This act was developed to provide you with minimum standards in preventing health hazards. All necessary measures should be taken to prevent health hazards from occurring, including those not specified by the act.

In this chapter, we will discuss some of the regulations put forward by the government that are applicable to eyelash extension artists. This is not a comprehensive guide to these regulations, and it does not serve to replace the government guidelines in full. You should also review the actual regulation – a link is found to the legislation in the resource section at the back of this book. Be aware that the government periodically updates regulation acts. Any updates that occur after this book is published can be sourced online through the government website.

General Operation Guidelines

The premises in which you are working should be maintained in a clean, sanitary, pest-free condition. Tables, counter tops and other furniture should be constructed of non-absorbent, easily cleanable material. In other words, don't decorate your space with that wall-to-wall hot pink shag rug, no matter how tempting it is, or how good it might look!

You must have a sink with hot and cold running water, dispensable soap and single-service towels available to both patrons and operators. Proper hand washing is the first step in preventing communicable disease transfer.

According to the act, you must also ensure that the space you are offering personal services from is entirely separate from any premise used for living or sleeping purposes, is away from any food storage or service, or other incompatible business, and is adequately lighted and ventilated for your particular service. This does not mean that you cannot operate your business from home. This means the space in your home from which you are offering this service should be completely separate from your living space. A small room, or area of a room, reserved specifically for your business can suffice in many cases.

You should ensure that you have the up-to-date Material Safety Data Sheets (MSDS) available for any hazardous products as provided by product suppliers. If you are purchasing your products directly from the manufacturer, ask them to supply these. If you are purchasing products from a retail outlet, the MSDS should also be available to you.

All towels, pillow coverings and other linens that come into contact with the a client must be thoroughly washed and dried in a clothes dryer at the hottest setting after each use. In many cases, using disposable linens may be more convenient, cost-effective and environmentally friendly.

Administering Drugs or Eye Drops

In British Columbia, it is considered an offense for a person to offer or to practice medicine while not being a registered primary healthcare provider. Healthcare professionals go through vigorous studies, practice, and completion of government implemented board exams, followed by continuing education, to achieve registration status.

If you are not a registered healthcare practitioner, you cannot administer drugs. This includes the administration of over the counter drugs like eye drops, Tylenol or Advil. The complete details on this subject can be reviewed in the Health Act's Personal Service Establishments Regulation and should be understood by every eyelash extension artist.

While it is an offense to offer drugs or medications to your clients, there is no harm in having unopened, non-prescription individual-use eye drops on hand, in case your client requests the same. You should not offer the client eye drops, but if they make the request you may give them unopened, over the counter products. It is imperative that the client opens the original packaging themselves and that they administer the drops on their own. Do not assist the client in drug administration, and do not allow multiple clients to use the same eye drop container.

If you offer your client any form of drug or medication, help administer any form of drug of medication, or allow the client to use a previously opened drug or medication, you may be held liable for any adverse reactions to the use of that drug or medication.

Equipment

Equipment, instruments and supplies should be constructed of durable materials and should be maintained in good repair. You should only use equipment that you are properly trained to handle. Any equipment or surface that comes into contact with exposed skin must be easily cleaned and must be disinfected before each use. Alternatively, approved single-use disposable materials may be used, and should be replaced before each new client. Tabletops should be disinfected between clients, and pillowcases should be washed, or discarded if they are disposable pillowcases. Tweezers and cosmetic scissors should be properly disinfected between each use, while items like micro brushes and cotton swabs should be discarded immediately after use.

Infection Control

The best way to prevent the spread of disease is to wash your hands well, before attending to any new client and then again after finishing with that client. While this is common knowledge among health professionals, and in some industries, many people still don't know how to properly wash their hands. The health act defines the proper hand washing procedure as follows:

1. Remove all jewelry.
2. Wet hands with warm, running water.
3. Apply liquid soap and lather well being sure to rub your hands vigorously as you wash them.
4. Wash all surfaces of the hands including
    a. Backs of hands
    b. Wrists
    c. Between the fingers
    d. Under the fingernails
5. Rinse hands well and then leave the water running.

6. Repeat steps 3 through 5.
7. Leaving water running, dry hands with a single-use towel.
8. Using the single use towel to avoid touching the tap, turn off the running water.

Sterilization & Disinfection

The equipment used for eyelash extension application, tweezers and cosmetic scissors, etc. are considered semi-critical items by our government. Semi-critical items are defined as those items that come into contact with mucous membranes, e.g. eyes, ears, nose, mouth, or any other body orifices, or skin that is not intact. These items must either be purchased sterile and then disposed of after a single use, or must be treated using high level disinfection before the first use, and after each consecutive use.

High-Level Disinfection

High-Level Disinfection is considered to destroy all microorganisms with the exception of some bacterial spores. While the government recognizes many methods of accomplishing this, the most applicable, financially obtainable, and convenient to the eyelash extension industry, is using a chemical sterilant. Chemical sterilization may only be used if precise controls on organic load, shelf life, contact time, temperature, and pH are managed. There are products that can be purchased for this specific purpose, like the PREempt CS20, or Barbicide that is often seen in salons. You can achieve high-level disinfection using some specific brands of household disinfecting bleach. The precise instructions for this will follow. When using products designed specifically for high-level disinfection, the manufacturer's directions must be followed at all times.

To accomplish high-level disinfection using any solution, the following steps should be followed:

1. Rinse items in hot water (cool water if blood-soiled).
2. Wash debris from items.
3. Place items in a disinfecting bath immediately after use.
4. Rinse.

5. Handle and store items so as to prevent contamination before next use.

High-Level Disinfection with Bleach

Fresh solution should be mixed once per day. Do not use this solution for multiple days in a row. The following instructions create a dilution, as mandated by the government of BC, for using household bleach to disinfect semi-critical items. Note that the bleach used must have a DIN (Health Canada's Drug Identification Number) and must indicate "HLD" (High Level Disinfectant) on the label. There is a web address in the Resource section at the back of this book that shares these details for an Ultra Clorox brand Disinfecting bleach that meets these requirements. In an instrument bath:

1. Add ½ cup household bleach to 4 cups water. For less total solution, add ⅛ cup bleach to 1 cup of water.
2. Leave instruments in bath for no less than 20 minutes.

Other Materials

Creams, lotions, powders and other cosmetics should be kept in clean, closed containers. These should either be individualized single-service package portions, or should be dispensed using a clean, single service spatula to remove the portion of the substance required.

Any fluids that come into contact with mucous membranes (like the eyeball) should be sterile. This means, if you intend to keep eye-drops or false tears on hand for your client's use (which is not necessary but is common in the eyelash extension industry), it must be packaged in sterile, single-use containers. You cannot allow multiple clients to use the same eye-drop bottle.

Personnel

Anyone who is providing personal services must practice acceptable personal hygiene. This includes proper washing of hands with soap and water before and after the service, and wearing clean outer garments. The provider should not smoke while providing the service. The provider must demonstrate competency in the use of equipment and in the methods for their field of practice. In other words, an eyelash extension artist must have the dexterity to manage tweezers with control and confidence before attempting to offer the service to the public.

If the provider has a known communicable disease, or open sores on the hands, they must observe proper infection control precautions including wearing protective barriers, like gloves.

Finally, any personal service provider should be familiar with the Health Act's Personal Service Establishments Regulation. The web address can be found in resource section at the back of the book.

Chapter Summary Points
- All efforts should be taken to prevent the spread of disease.
- Only registered healthcare professionals may offer or administer drugs, including over the counter eye drops.
- Eyelash extension artists must be familiar with and abide by the Health Act's Personal Service Establishments Regulation.
- The premises in which the service is provided must be easily cleaned and suitable for the service being provided.
- Equipment must be either single use, or properly cleaned and disinfected prior to each use.
- Personnel must follow basic personal hygiene and be familiar with proper hand washing procedures.

Definitions

Personal service establishment	a place in which a person provides a personal service to or on the body of another person
Sanitary	hygienic and clean
Liable	responsible by law; legally answerable
Communicable disease	an illness caused by an infectious agent or its toxic products

7. Safety & First Aid

In order to work with the public you should have valid first aid certification received through a recognized first aid course provider in your area. In addition to the standard first aid training that anyone working with the public should have, there are circumstances that are more likely to occur during an eyelash extension service than in other industries. Here, we'll cover basic first aid for situations you may encounter specific to this industry. Keep in mind that if the product manufacturer supplied first aid instructions with the product you are using, those instructions should be followed. If you find there are instructions listed here that conflict with, or contradict, the first aid instructions you have been taught during a recognized first aid certification course, the certification course instructions should be followed.

Eyelash extension artists use a number of chemicals and other irritants in close proximity to their client's eyes. Eyelash cleansers and primers will often contain chemicals, including ethyl alcohol and isopropyl alcohol, or a combination of both. Eyelash adhesives are cyanoacrylate glues. These are strong glues that are used in household repairs and in medical settings. Eyelash adhesive removers often contain very strong chemical solvents. Many people are sensitive to, or have allergies to, these types of ingredients, and even those who don't have sensitivities may suffer serious side effects if the products are mismanaged. For these reasons, you must be well versed in using these products, and your clients should be aware of the chemical nature of these products, and any potential adverse effects prior to you beginning the application process. In addition, you should be capable of competently dealing with any situation requiring first aid.

General Product Precautions

None of the products used should ever come into contact with the eyes, or touch the client's skin. The under eyelids and eyelashes should be protected with a barrier, and the client's eyes should stay closed for the duration of the service to prevent product or product fumes from seeping into the eye socket and onto the surface of the eyeball. Eyelash extensions are to be bonded to the eyelash itself, millimeters from the skin and they should not touch the eyelid. You must fan the eyelashes at the end of the service and before your client opens their eyes, to dissipate any remaining fumes. During a full eyelash extension removal, your client should be seated in an upright position, as gel removers tend to liquefy as they work and sitting upright helps prevent remover leakage into the eye. We'll discuss this further as we cover the application and removal processes. You should only offer eyelash extension application service in a well-ventilated area, and you should keep all products out of the reach of children. Eyelash extensions and application products are all flammable. Your client should be forewarned to keep eyelash extensions away from heat exposure, including that of lighting a cigarette or a BBQ.

Cyanoacrylate Cautions

Cyanoacrylate glues are known to have an exothermic reaction with cotton, wool & leather. This means when cyanoacrylate glues are combined with such things, the reaction creates heat, smoke and even spontaneous combustion. It is imperative that you do not use micro brushes, cotton swabs, or wipes on glue that has not yet dried and set. Once the glue has set, no chemical reaction should occur.

In addition to being exothermic, cyanoacrylate is a toxic vapor. You should take every effort to protect yourself and your clients from inhalation. At the very least, wear a mask that is suitable for filtering chemical fumes and keep your glue away from your client's nose and mouth. Some artists will purchase chemical fume extractors, and there are some places in the world where these units are necessary by law in order to work with adhesives. Note that a regular medical mask is not enough to filter chemical fumes.

Acute symptoms may not appear immediately with exposure to the fumes, however, prolonged breathing of cyanoacrylate fumes can lead to serious respiratory dysfunctions and illnesses. Taking appropriate precautions right from the start will help ensure your career, as an eyelash extension artist, is a long and healthy one!

First Aid for Product Eye Contact

If any of the products used get into your client's eyes, and the eyelids will still easily open you should:

1. Flush the open eyes with running water or a sterile saline solution created specifically for the eyes, for a minimum of 15 minutes.
2. If redness, irritation or any symptoms persist, contact a physician immediately.

If eyelids are bonded closed:

1. Do NOT force open the eyes.
2. Flush eye with running water for a minimum of 15 minutes. Cover with sterile, dry bandages.
3. Seek immediate medical attention.
4. The eye should open in time without further action.
5. If burns occur, they are to be treated as thermal (heat or fire) burns.

If first aid attempts resolve immediate symptoms, but further redness or irritation occurs, the client should seek medical attention.

First Aid for Product Skin Contact

Many of the products used in eyelash extension application may irritate sensitive skin. If any of the products used come into contact with the skin you should:

1. Remove any contaminated clothing and wipe any excess product off the skin.
2. Wash exposed area thoroughly with soap and water.
3. Flush with running water for at least 15 minutes.
4. If redness, itching, a burning sensation, or any symptoms develop, seek medical attention.

First Aid for Product Inhalation

The vapors of many of these products may cause headache, nausea and irritation to throat and lungs. Prolonged and repeated exposure may cause non-allergic asthma-like symptoms in some individuals. If there are any signs of adverse reactions to the inhalation of these products you should:

1. Evacuate the area and prevent further exposure to vapors.
2. If the affected person becomes unconscious call 911, or the emergency medical service in your area.
3. If breathing becomes difficult, administer oxygen (if available).
4. If breathing stops, administer CPR until emergency response arrives, or the person starts breathing again.

If first aid attempts resolve immediate symptoms, but further irritation occurs, seek medical attention.

First Aid for Product Ingestion

While ingestion may be unlikely you should still be prepared to respond should it occur. If any of the products used are ingested, and there are no apparent symptoms, you should:

1. Contact your local poison control center. In British Columbia the phone number is 1-800-567-8911. Keep this number, or the number for poison control in your area, in an easily accessible place near where you are working.

If any of the products are ingested and there are symptoms you should:

1. Seek immediate medical attention.

If first aid attempts resolve immediate symptoms, but further symptoms occur at a later time, seek medical attention.

Chapter Summary Points

- Eyelash extension artists should be certified in basic first aid, and should be familiar with basic first aid surrounding the chemical products they are using.

- Product in eyes or on skin should be flushed with running water for a minimum of 15 minutes.
- If the product is inhaled you must move to a well-ventilated area with clean air.
- If loss of consciousness occurs, call 911 or the emergency medical services in your area immediately.
- In British Columbia the Poison Control Centre phone number is 1-800-567-8911.
- If symptoms persist post first aid, or when in doubt, seek medical attention.

Definitions

Ethyl alcohol	is the principal type of alcohol found in alcoholic beverages, produced by the fermentation of sugars by yeasts
Isopropyl alcohol	a liquid alcohol, used as a solvent and in the industrial production of acetone
Cyanoacrylate	any of a class of compounds that are cyanide derivatives of acrylates. They are easily polymerized and are used to make quick-setting adhesives
Dissipate	disperse or scatter
Spontaneous combustion	the bursting into flame of a mass of material as a result of chemical reactions within the substance, without the addition of heat from an external source
Saline solution	a sterile solution of sodium chloride in water

8. Professional Eyelash Extension Products

There are a number of products specific to eyelash extensions that an artist will want to have on hand. Here, we'll discuss the items that are necessary for application, as well as some of the other optional tools available.

Tweezers

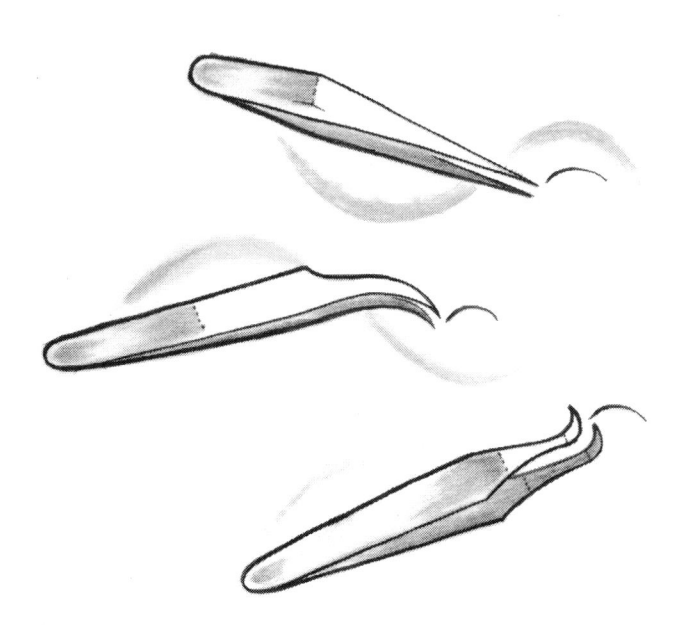

Tweezers are arguably an eyelash extension artist's most important tool. High quality precision tweezers are expensive, with the cost sometimes ranging into the hundreds of dollars. The style and shape of tweezers used, while distinctly individual to the artist, should have some similarities dependent on the tweezers' purpose. You will need at least two, possibly three, different types of tweezers: a straight or bent-nosed set of tweezers for separating and isolating eyelashes, a curved-nosed set of tweezers for picking up eyelash extensions, dipping them in glue, and then applying them to the natural lash that you have isolated with the straight-nosed pair of tweezers, and the third type of tweezers designed specifically for building eyelash extension fans. We will discuss building lash fans later. Now, just note that the tweezers used for creating fans are built with precision, and have the most contact area near the tips to allow for manipulation of individual single eyelash extensions.

Fans & Puffers

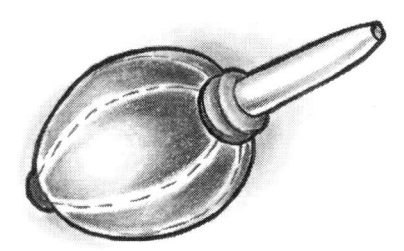

Throughout the eyelash extension application process there are times when the eyelashes must be dried. This can be achieved with an eyelash puffer, or a rechargeable portable electric fan. Another option is using a small, low voltage, extremely low or cold temperature hair dryer.

Glue Carriers

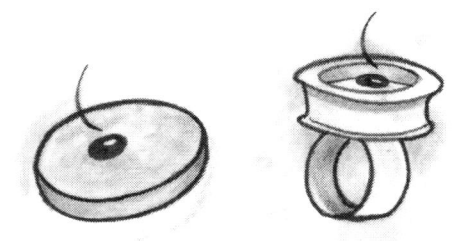

During the application process, the eyelash extensions are dipped a millimeter or two, into a drop of glue. The drop of glue is often placed on a glass or jade stone or ring, or in a plastic ring cup designed specifically for this purpose.

Lash Rings or Bulbs

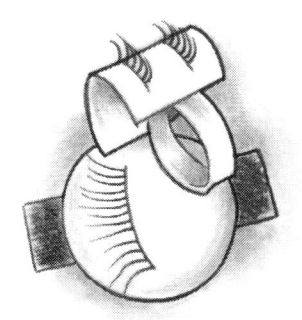

While not necessary for lash extension application, some artists prefer to use a lash ring or dome. These are designed in a round, convex shape, to separate the lashes, which make them easier to pluck individually or to fan into groups for volume applications. Using half an empty vending machine capsule, half a plastic ball or a dome-shaped paperweight may achieve the same results without the added expense.

Under Eyelid Lash Barriers

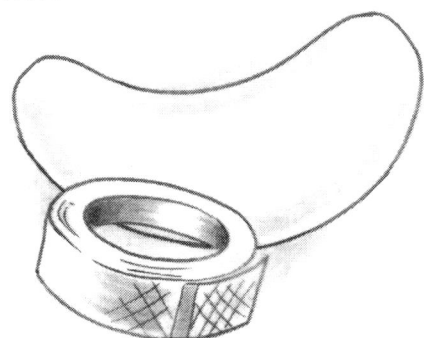

Gel pads, stickers, and medical tape, are all used as barriers to protect the under eyelid and lashes during the eyelash extension application process. Gel pads, while the most expensive option, will moisturize and sooth the skin under your client's eyes while you work. Stickers and medical tape should not be too sticky or tacky as they may pull out the lower eyelashes when removed. And whatever your preference is, you should not use medical tape alone as it does not cover enough surface area to suffice as a protective barrier.

Cosmetic Scissors

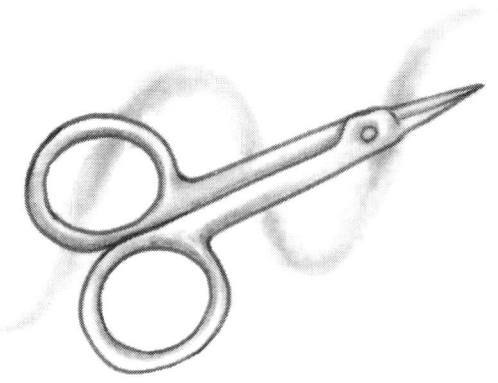

Cosmetic scissors are used as a last resort if two or more eyelash extensions have been stuck together in a T-shape and cannot be peeled apart by other means. Note that both natural lashes and eyelash extensions are tapered and, as such, cutting them will leave an unnatural-looking blunt edge. If a natural lash is cut, an extension should be applied to it immediately. An eyelash extension artist will only cut lashes if absolutely necessary.

Disposable Eyelash Wands

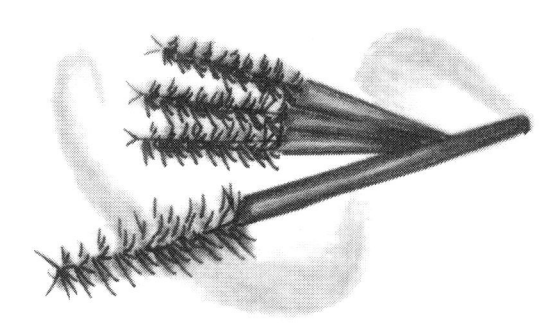

Disposable eyelash wands are used to disperse the eyelash primer at the beginning of an application, and to brush the natural lashes and the eyelash extensions throughout and after the application process. At the end of the application, these wands should be given to the client so they can continue to brush their extensions on their own after the appointment. You should never use the same eyelash wand on multiple clients.

Micro Brushes

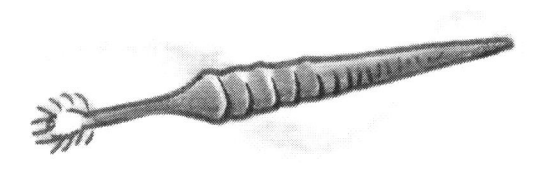

Micro brushes are specifically designed to be lint free and are used to apply cleansers, primer, or pre-treatment to the eyelashes at the start of the application process. They are also used for spot applying a gel or cream adhesive remover, if just one eyelash extension needs to be removed. Note that the tips of these should never come in contact with wet glue.

Cotton Swabs

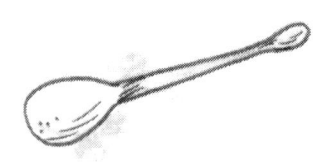

Cotton swabs are used with a filtered or distilled water to wash the lashes when necessary. Note that the tips of these should never come in contact with wet glue.

Eyelash Extensions

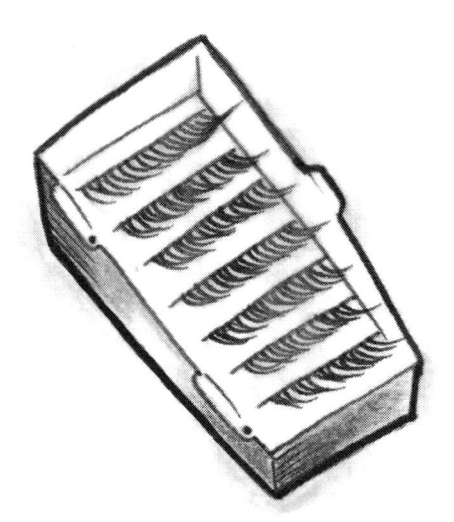

Eyelash extensions are made of silk, mink hair or a synthetic version of either of these. They come in multiple shapes, lengths, thicknesses and even colors. Thickness is measured at the base of the eyelash extension, and like natural eyelashes the extensions are tapered to a fine point. They are sold in tubs or in trays, with varying numbers of rows, sometimes with mixed lengths in the same tray. You can buy individual lashes or pre-fanned lashes. The lash extension choice you make for each new client will affect the finished look you create. The combined use of some of the many variations available allow for many different finished looks. The eyelash extensions you choose to use is where the creativity of this job really starts!

By far the most common material that lashes are made of is a synthetic silk or synthetic mink. More often than not, the words 'silk' or 'mink' actually refer to the appearance of the lashes, and not the actual material they are made from. Lashes referred to as silk will have a matte coloring, while lashes referred to as mink will be shinier. Synthetic lashes will melt when in contact with extreme temperatures. Thicker lashes give eyelash extensions a glamorous, fully made-up finished look. They will have a false plastic-like feel to them when applied if they are too thick. Extensions described as silk can be expensive. They tend to have a duller, more natural look and feel when applied.

Mink lashes are made of real mink hair and are the most expensive, as well as the most natural looking and feeling lash extensions available. They are also the least used in the west, due to animal cruelty concerns and the fact that they do not maintain their curl.

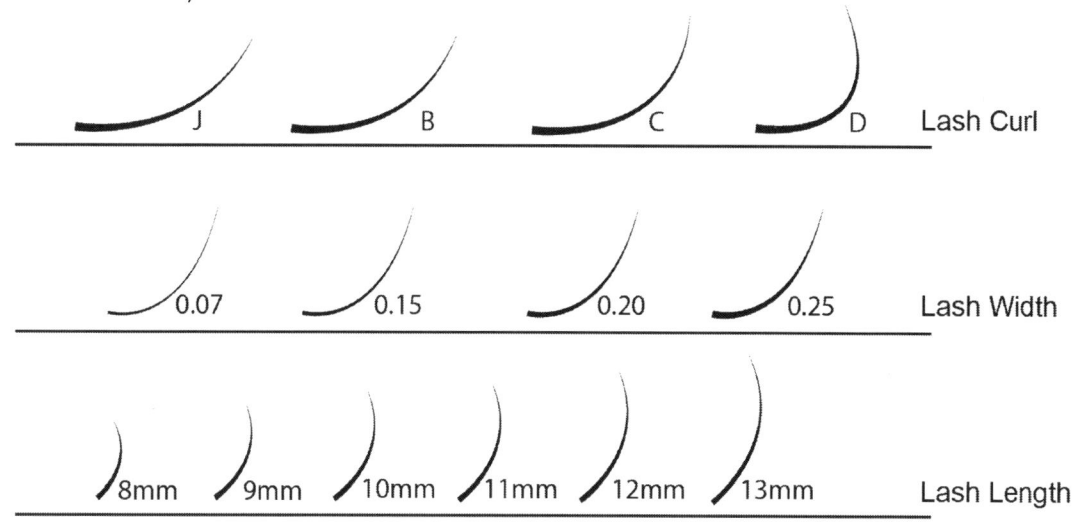

J	B	C	D	Lash Curl
0.07	0.15	0.20	0.25	Lash Width
8mm	9mm	10mm	11mm	12mm	13mm	Lash Length

The most common curl-shapes, widths, and lengths of lashes are illustrated in the above diagram. The diagram is not to scale. Also available are L, L+ and U curls. These are extreme curls, the L variations having an acute angle in them to create something of an L-shape rather than a curl, and the U-curl are so extreme as to actually look like the letter U.

In western practise the most common shapes used are J, B & C curls, that range from 8mm to 12mm long, and are 0.15mm thick for a classic extension set, and 0.07mm for a volume set. Lash extensions are available as small as 0.05mm thick through 0.10mm mid-sized, and as large as 0.25mm thickness. We will discuss lash selection further when we discuss the application processes.

Relatively new on the market are Ellipse or Flat extensions. These lashes are not cylindrical in shape, but instead are flat at the base. It makes for a lighter, yet wider looking lash and some eyelash extension artists feel it makes the application process easier. The below diagram illustrates what the difference between a classic and a flat extension looks like, at the base, while attached to a natural eyelash.

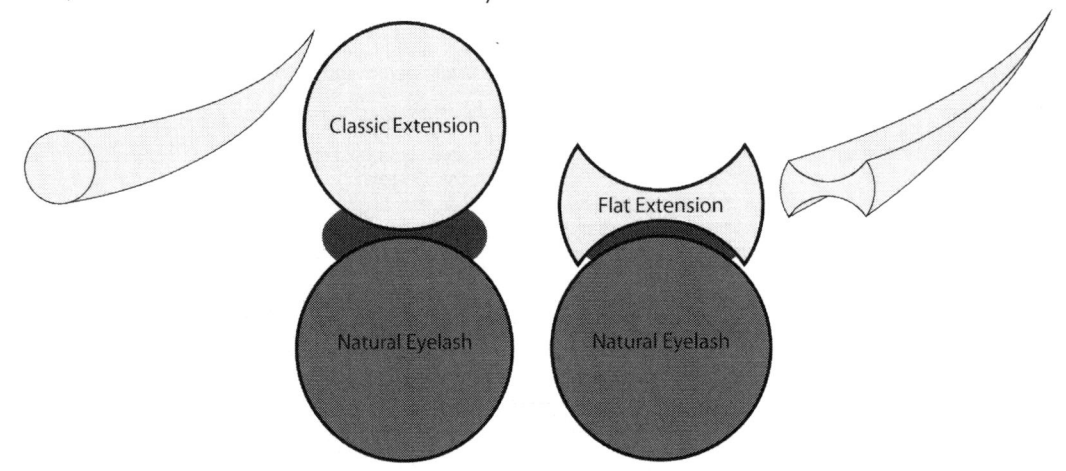

You can visualize how a flat lash with the same diameter of a classic lash will actually be thinner, and as such will weigh less than a classic lash. This is worth considering when you're selecting the best extension for your client based on their natural lashes. We will further discuss lash selection later.

In purchasing your eyelash extensions, in addition to material, shape and size, you'll also want to consider the packaging. Tubs of single loose lashes may have more lashes per package, but are not organized, and as such, it may take you longer to select and pick up the lash you wish to use in an appropriate manner during the application process. Tray lashes, while easiest to pick up by the tapered tip of the lash as necessary for application, are adhered to the tray with a low-tack adhesive strip. If the adhesive used in the tray is too strong, as seen in many cheap variety lash extensions, the lash will be difficult to remove from the tray, and bits of tray adhesive may remain on it. This causes an excess amount of eyelash glue to remain on the extension, and will result in a weaker adhesive bond with the natural lash, more weight to be applied to each individual natural eyelash, and a messier finished look.

Eyelash Cleansers & Primers

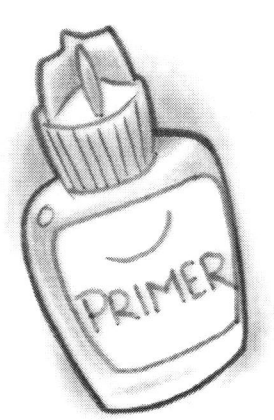

Eyelash cleansers and primers are used to clean and prepare the natural eyelash for extension application. Makeup particles and natural oils found on the eyelashes will reduce the staying power of the adhesive. If the eyelashes are not completely cleaned at the start of the application, the bond will not set as strong as it otherwise would, and your extensions will not last.

Cleansers are usually made of a mix of water and ethyl and/or isopropyl alcohol. This combination breaks down oils and effectively works to thoroughly clean the lashes of excess proteins. Cleansers are found in the form of protein remover wipes, which are pre-moistened wipes, or in solution form.

Primers are usually made of water, polyvinylpyrrolidone (PVP), polyacrylate & ethanol, and work to dry and prepare the eyelash surface for the best possible bonding with the adhesive. Primers, with ethanol, serve to clean the lashes as well. If the client has clean eyelashes to start with, a primer will work to clean and prepare the natural eyelashes for the application process. You can make your own eyelash cleanser/primer by mixing 6 parts distilled water with 4 parts medical grade isopropyl or ethyl alcohol.

Eyelash Extension Glue

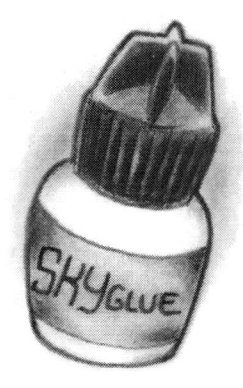

Eyelash extension glue is often the most expensive disposable tool in an eyelash extension artist's kit. Made of a cyanoacrylate, the exact same component that gives super glue it's instant bonding power, this glue is incredibly strong, fast acting, and toxic. In this section, we'll learn why it's imperative that your eyelash extension is attached only to your client's eyelash, and not to allow the glue to touch your, or your client's, skin.

There are 4 common variations of cyanoacrylate glues, each with different chemical structures.

Methyl-Cyanoacrylate   Ethyl-Cyanoacrylate   Butyl-Cyanoacrylate   Octyl-Cyanoacrylate

Each of these is created through a condensation process that combines both cyano-acetate and formaldehyde. What remains after the process is refined with stabilizers, and other additives. Formaldehyde will no longer be present in the finished product. Methyl-Cyanoacrylate and Ethyl-Cyanoacrylate are sold in unsterile, reusable packaging like Krazy Glue. Both Super Glue and professional eyelash extension glues are most often created with Ethyl-Cyanoacrylate.

For the eyelash application process, we only use small drops at any given time, however, it's important to be familiar with the potential side effects. All eyelash glue is histotoxic (toxic to tissue) and contains known carcinogens. It is imperative that the glue does not touch the skin, or come into contact with the eye. The vapor is irritating to the eyes, skin, mucous membranes, and respiratory tract. These chemicals may cause sensitization by inhalation, and over exposure can lead to narcotic effects, headaches, dizziness, and vomiting. You must keep your glues out of the reach of children and be familiar with first aid as previously discussed. Eyelash glues can be stored for up to a year in a cool, dark place if unopened. Once opened, with proper use and storage, they have a shelf life of 3 to 6 months.

Butyl-Cyanoacrylate is considered medical grade glue and is sold as Vetbond only to licensed veterinarians in British Columbia. Octyl-Cyanoacrylate is also considered medical grade glue and is sold as Dermabond. This is also sold only to medical professionals in British Columbia, and at prices reaching more than $70 USD for a single-use 0.7ml container. Butyl-Cyanoacrylate and Octyl-Cyanoacrylate cure slower than Ethyl-Cyanoacrylate and Methyl-Cyanoacrylate. Medical grade cyanoacrylate glues are still widely used in the veterinary industry in place of stitches for skin bonding, but are used less in a human medical setting, due to the discovery of their histotoxic nature. They still serve a place for emergency use in first aid kits, especially in remote wilderness settings. Medical grade glues are sold only in single-use sterile containers.

There are eyelash extension artists who claim to use medical grade glue for their extensions and there are brands that claim to sell medical grade adhesives. With medical grade glues being so difficult to get in British Columbia, with longer curing times and sold only in single-use containers at such high prices, I question whether or not those statements are factual, or are based on the misleading claims made by the product manufacturers or sales people. What's considered medical grade in the manufacturer's country is not necessarily considered medical grade by western standards. If you are hoping to use a medical grade cyanoacrylate adhesive, I recommend you speak to a pharmacist, chemist or other medical professional in your country, and not a sales person who is pushing a product on you under false claims.

When purchasing eyelash glues, many marketing statements are made about the setting time. The way cyanoacrylate glues bond depends on the amount of spreading the glue can do in a given time between two surfaces. The more it can spread, the quicker it will bond. Therefore, the more liquid your glue is, the faster it will set. Thickened glue will spread slower and as result it will set slower. On contact with water, cyanoacrylate glues spread instantly, causing an instant drying and setting. All cyanoacrylate glues will set in just a few seconds with proper use.

Eyelash Adhesive Removers

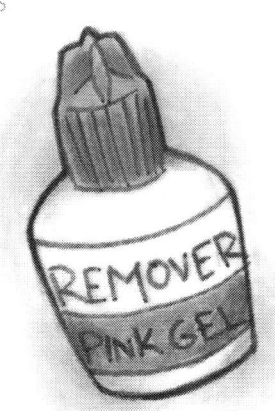

As you can imagine, anything that serves to break down the bonds of cyanoacrylate glue must be incredibly potent. This is certainly the case with eyelash adhesive removers. The chemicals found in these removers include, but are not limited to, propylene carbonate, poly ethylene glycol, and 2-oxotetrahydrofuran.

Adhesive removers may cause eye irritation, skin irritation, digestive tract disturbances if ingested, and respiratory tract irritation if inhaled. There is evidence of carcinogenic effects from these ingredients. Like the eyelash glue, gel remover must be used sparingly, should not come into contact with the skin or eyes of yourself or your client. Be familiar with proper first aid responses should contact occur. Always clean the eye area thoroughly after use, and then even have the client wash their face, if possible. If the use of a remover can be avoided, it is best to do so.

You should have gel, cream, or both removers on hand in case of emergency. An example emergency situation would be your client suffering a severe allergic reaction to the eyelash extensions or glue, and needing them removed immediately, before a medical professional can treat the reaction. Should removal be necessary under these circumstances, take every precaution possible to prevent the leakage of gel remover onto your clients skin or into your client's eye. This will be discussed further when we discuss removal procedures.

Nano Misters

Nano misters are sometimes referred to as facial misters or vaporizers. They are electric gadgets that turn water into an extremely fine mist. They are perfect for use at the end of the eyelash extension application process to set the adhesive. This is sometimes unnecessary, depending on the humidity of the environment that the lash artist is working in, but is a good idea in the west. At the very least, use of the Nano Mister will ensure that there are no fumes lingering around the eyes when the client is ready to open their eyes.

Thermometers & Hygrometers

Thermometers are used to measure room temperature and hygrometers are used to measure humidity. Both temperature and humidity play an important role in how eyelash extension adhesive works. The higher the humidity, the quicker your glue will set. This is extremely important in Russian Volume applications, which we will discuss later.

Chapter Summary Points

- There are a number of products and tools specific to an eyelash extension artist.
- Many of the products necessary are toxic and should only be used with extreme caution.
- The tools necessary to apply eyelash extensions include tweezers, under-eye barriers, micro brushes, disposable wands, an eyelash cleanser or primer, adhesive, adhesive remover, an eyelash fan or puffer, and the eyelash extensions.

- Other accessories are available to make your job as an eyelash extension artist easier.

Definitions

Precision	the quality, condition, or fact of being exact and accurate
Formaldehyde	a colorless pungent gas in solution made by oxidizing methanol
Histotoxic	poisonous to tissues
Carcinogen	a substance capable of causing cancer in living tissue

9. Client Consultation & Consent

Before working on your client, they should fill out an intake form that makes you aware of any health concerns, allergies or other reasons why you may not proceed, or would proceed only with extreme caution, in applying eyelash extensions. There is a sample intake form in the appendix of this book that you may wish to modify and use.

For your safety, and the safety of your clients, you must also be sure to start every eyelash extension appointment with a short consultation during which you will advise a new client, or remind a returning client, of some of the more pertinent details of the application process, and the importance of their after care. This conversation should cover specific client considerations, including the things they may not think of on their own. You should discuss the application process and any new products you are using, potential risks and side effects, and after care instructions. You should determine that your client has no allergies or sensitivities to the products you are using. You should also get an idea of the style of lashes the client is aiming for, and make your extension size and shape choices based on the client's feedback. New clients should always be offered a patch test at least 24-48 hours prior to the actual application, and all clients should sign a liability waiver before you start working on them. There is a sample liability form found with the intake form in the appendix of this book.

In addition to having a completed intake form and a signed liability waiver on file for each client, you may wish to keep a short record of appointment notes on file. This can serve as a reminder of each appointment date, and each appointment specific lash look goals, as well as the exact extensions you used to achieve the look. This may be beneficial for future appointments when clients ask for, "that same style you did last time." Often, you end up seeing so many clients you simply won't remember what style you last created for them! I also like to keep a photo history record of before and after pictures for each and every client that I work with.

Client Considerations

Before you begin working on a client, they should be aware of the costs involved in maintaining their eyelash extensions with fill appointments and the cost of removal appointments, should removal be necessary. The importance of not rubbing or pulling on extensions should be stressed, and they should be advised that it takes up to 8 weeks for a hair to grow back if the natural lashes are prematurely pulled out. The client should be informed of the natural growth cycle of eyelashes, to prevent panicking if a few lashes extensions fall out soon after being applied. Once extensions are applied, the lashes are bigger and more noticeable, even as they fall out! Your client will want to consider any potential reaction, especially if they are having eyelash extensions applied for the first time for a special occasion. Eyelash extensions should be applied far enough in advance of any special occasion that any possible side effect, like sensitivities leading to conjunctivitis or puffiness can be resolved before their event.

Client's Daily Activity & After Care

Eyelash extension aftercare is important in maintaining a clean, healthy look and for increasing the longevity of the extensions. For the first few hours immediately after the application your client should not touch the eyelashes with their hands, as the oils in their hands may degrade the glue. Some eyelash extension artists will stress the importance of not getting the extensions wet at all for the first 2 to 48 hours. This is contrary to the scientific evidence of how cyanoacrylate glues work on a chemical level. As we previously discussed, water instantly sets eyelash extension glue. In my practice, I ask clients to wash their face as normal after their extensions are applied, and my work is known for its longevity just the same.

You should get an idea of the client's daily activities and advise accordingly. If your client is a swimmer or a hot yoga enthusiast, or anyone who spends large amounts of time in a hot, moist or wet environment, they should be aware that prolonged time in these environments might lead to premature breakdown of the eyelash adhesive. This will result in a reduced staying power and a more frequent need for fill appointments.

Bursts of extreme heat will melt or burn the extensions and the natural eyelashes, and possibly lead to injury, so caution should be given to smokers, or BBQ enthusiasts! Clients should be advised not to curl their eyelashes, using a heated or manual curler. Curlers of any type may damage the extensions by heat, or cause the manual breakdown of the adhesive bond, and in some cases, even pull out the lashes. If curl is desired, a curled eyelash extension should be used during the eyelash extension application.

While most people find the eyelash extensions eliminate the need for eye makeup, there are some who still wish to apply mascara, shadows and liners. Your client should never use waterproof mascara on eyelash extensions, or any oil based creams, liners or shadows. Water-based, water soluble mascara should be applied only to the tips of the eyelash extensions, avoiding the base where the extension is glued to the natural lash. Makeup should be cleaned off thoroughly with an oil-free cleanser at least once every 24-hours. Makeup that is not cleaned properly will adhere to the eyelash glue, possibly causing the partial breakdown and resetting of glue and a clump of a glue-like substance that holds multiple lashes together. Remind your client that eyelashes grow at different speeds and this clump may lead to the premature plucking of their natural lashes, and permanent damage to the hair follicle. Some oily oil-based products will slowly break down the eyelash extension adhesive and lead to premature falling out of the extensions.

In addition to discussing the aftercare with your client verbally, a comprehensive bulleted list of aftercare instructions that you can copy, print out, and give to your clients can be found in the appendix of this book.

Cleansing & Brushing Lash Extensions

During the eyelash extension application process, an eyelash extension artist uses an eyelash wand to brush the lashes and the lash extensions. This brush should be given to the client at the end of the appointment so they can brush their own eyelash extensions regularly, to help them maintain the eyelash shape in-between appointments. Having an eyelash wand prevents the client from using their fingers to touch the lashes, which otherwise reduces the extensions life through exposure to the natural oils found on the hands.

Mild Eyelash Cleanser

Clients can purchase eyelash shampoo, that are specially formulated for the use on the eyelashes or they can use their regular face wash, assuming it is oil free. They may also create their own gentle eyelash shampoo using a basic formula of 1 part no-tear baby wash and 2 parts filtered or distilled water. This is best used in a foaming dispenser. Note that there are old wives tales that claim no-tear shampoos block tear ducts or have a chemical anesthetic numbing agent added to them to prevent tearing. These claims are not true, nor are they based on any scientific facts. No-tear shampoos simply contain less surfactants (short for "surface active agents") than regular soaps and shampoos. Surfactants are the powerful cleansing agents used to cleanse oils and grit from the scalp and skin and can be irritating to the eyes. By using less of them, the cleansing power is reduced and there is less irritation. Baby shampoos are gentle, less effective but less irritating cleansers that are perfectly suitable for cleansing eyelash extensions. In fact, the ingredients found in baby shampoos are very similar to those found in eyelash shampoos!

Chapter Summary Points

- In addition to having a completed intake form from you client, before you begin working on them you should have a conversation, explaining the process, the tools and the chemicals you are about to use on them.
- You client should understand the procedure and the potential risks involved, and they should agree to the process before you begin.
- Informed consent is your legal obligation, and is in your best interest, as well as the best interest of your client.

Definitions

Longevity	long existence or service
Surfactant	a substance that tends to reduce the surface tension of a liquid in which it is dissolved

10. Station Set Up

Setting up your workstation before your client arrives leads to a smooth application appointment and a professional overall feel to the services you offer. Your workstation should include a bed, chaise, or table that your client can lay down on, on their back, so that you can easily access the eyelashes from above their head while they recline. A portable massage table works great for this! Your workstation should include a comfortable, adjustable chair for you to sit on while you work, a table or cart with all your supplies and an appropriate light source – preferably from above with a natural daylight-emitting bulb. Selecting a light bulb that simulates natural daylight will reduce strain on your eyes.

Lashing Environment Temperature & Humidity

We already discussed how eyelash extension glues are created with cyanoacrylate and do not dry, so much as cure. The speed at which they cure depends on the water content in the air (humidity), as well as the temperature of the space you are working in. The optimal temperature for eyelash extension adhesive to set in an appropriate amount of time, for most eyelash adhesives, is between 19°C and 24°C (66°F – 75.2°F), and the optimal humidity range is between 45% and 55%. This will vary slightly depending on the extension glue that you use.

The environment you work in should be controlled in order to maintain an ideal environment for your glue to set in an appropriate amount of time. For this reason, it is not ideal for eyelash extension artists to offer mobile services. This may mean you must invest in a good thermometer and hygrometer, especially if you are having trouble with lash retention or your glue setting. And some eyelash extension artists, who live and work in extreme environments, will go as far as investing in room dehydrators and air conditioners. Luckily, for those of us on the west coast of Canada, this does not seem necessary.

Client Comfort

In order to ensure your client's comfort you should start every appointment by making sure they are ready to lie down and close their eyes for a prolonged time. You may want to offer them a glass of water before you start, and you should invite them to use the bathroom. While it is possible to take a break mid-application to allow for use of the bathroom, if necessary, it is easier for them to simply go in advance if possible.

The table or chaise that you are using can be made more comfortable for your client with the placement of a few pillows, one small one for the neck and head, and a larger bolster-like pillow for below the knees. If you offer your client a pillow for the neck and head, make sure the bulk of it is under the client's neck so that the chin is pointed up towards the ceiling and the lashes are on an angle away from the under-eyelid. Failing to do this will result in lashes being glued to the protective under-eye barrier. C-shaped travel pillows positioned under the clients neck work well for this. A knee pillow, placed under your client's knees while they lay on their back, will lessen torquing of the hips and helps reduce low back stress, which would otherwise cause discomfort. Discomfort may cause your client to make adjustment movements while you work.

You may also choose to leave a throw or blanket on the table, especially if you're working in a cool environment. Many clients do doze off or fall asleep during the application process, which makes the application easier for you. Why not make it easier for them to do so?

Artist's Comfort

The application process can take 2 to 3 hours to complete. It is important that you as the artist are also comfortable. You should be able to adjust the height of the chair you are working on as necessary so that throughout the application your back is maintained in an upright, straight position. Slumping over while you work may seem easiest at first, but will lead to back ache if too much time is spent in this position. Your knees should be able to rest under the table or chaise in front of you, under your client's head as it rests on the table. Your light source should come from above or another angle so that your hands will not cast a shadow on the eyelashes as you work.

Your client's movement may make the application process more difficult and more uncomfortable for you. When we speak, our faces subconsciously create expressions to match what we're saying, or the feelings we are trying to express. Eye movement, even when the eyes are closed is often a huge part of these facial expressions. It's ok to ask your client to keep the amount of chatting to a minimum while you work. Just be sure to ask them politely and to explain that talking leads to eye movement, which makes it more difficult for you to work with precision. Most clients understand this and want you to do the best possible job on them.

Lash, glue, and other tool placement, will be unique to you, and it may take a while for you to figure out what works best. If you are using lash and glue rings, you will place these on the finger(s) of your lash separating hand (usually the left hand for right-handed people). Lashes and glue may also be kept on the table to the right of your client's head if you are right-handed, or to the left if you are left-handed. Placing your working materials close to your client's head makes it easier for you to access while you work. Some eyelash extension artists will use a piece of double-sided tape to hold lashes on the back of their hand while they work. This is all totally up to you. Practice and you'll figure out what set up works best!

Tools & Supplies

Before your client arrives, you should have your workstation set up, with all your tools disinfected, and all of your supplies in place so that you are ready to begin working. The below items should be readily available at your work station:

- Medical tape, under-eye gel pads and/or stickers
- Eyelash extensions
- Glue ring, stone, plate or other glue carrier
- Eyelash primer
- Eyelash adhesive
- Adhesive remover
- Sterilized tweezers
- Sterilized cosmetic scissors
- Sanding file (nail file used to sand any glue off your tweezers if necessary)

- Acetone (used to clean any glue off your tweezers if necessary – you must rinse tweezers with water after dipping in acetone, prior to using them again on your clients eyes!)
- Disinfectant wipes or solution (for use in case you drop your tweezers on the ground while applying the eyelash extensions)
- Disposable eyelash wands
- Micro brushes
- Cotton swabs
- Filtered or distilled water
- Cotton balls or pads
- Eyelash dryer or puffer
- Petroleum jelly
- Nano Mister (if using)
- Hand mirror

Chapter Summary Points

- The optimal temperature for eyelash extension adhesive to set in an appropriate amount of time is said to be between 19°C and 24°C (66°F and 75.2°F), and the optimal humidity range is between 45% and 55%.
- You should set up your workstation before your client arrives to help maintain a professional environment.
- Making sure your client is comfortable will make your job easier because they will fidget less while you work.
- Make sure you are comfortable while you work, even if this means asking your client not to talk. Just be sure to ask politely and to explain why!
- Set up a workstation with lighting that is appropriate for your body, to prevent future eyestrain and back aches.

Definitions

Torque	to apply torque or a twisting force to (an object)
Hygrometer	an instrument for measuring the humidity of the air

11. Eyelash Extension Application

Now that we've looked at our station set up, let's look at the actual application process. It's important to note that the information contained in this book is not meant to replace hands-on learning. For proper application technique, you should take a hands-on course with a qualified instructor where you will get the opportunity to practice and be critiqued on your skills.

The application process is almost identical for a classic eyelash extension set, a volume extension set, or a Russian volume extension set. The difference is in what we are attaching to the isolated natural eyelash. We'll first cover application of classic extension set and then we will discuss what makes a volume, or Russian Volume set, different.

Selecting Safe Extension Lengths, Widths & Weights

A good eyelash extension artist will have a selection of extensions available to them because they are aware that their selections are limited by the client's natural lash. For the average person, and the majority of eyelash extension clients, your safest classic extension width is 0.15mm. For the rare client with extremely thick and strong natural lashes, you may choose to apply 0.18mm or even 0.20mm lashes. While thicker extensions than 0.20mm are available, it is extremely rare to find a client with suitable natural lashes for them. Many reputable lash extension shops will not even carry larger extensions for this reason. For clients who present with thinner, weaker natural lashes, you should choose a width of 0.10mm to 0.12mm.

For a classic, somewhat natural look set using 0.15mm width extensions, you may extend the natural lashes 2-3mm beyond the natural eyelash length. For a fuller more dramatic look, it may be safe to extend the natural lashes as much as 3-4mm, depending of course on the strength of the natural lashes to begin with. The thinner the extension width you choose, the safer it is to apply a longer extension. Flat extensions are not as heavy as classic extensions and as such, you may be able to apply thicker width, longer extensions using them than you would be able to apply using classic extensions. You will need to make an informed decision as to the lash capabilities depending on each client's natural lashes.

The reality is there is no set of rules as to how to select the correct eyelash extension for your client and each instructor will advise on something different. We all share the common goal of not causing damage to the client's natural lashes. In order to ensure that, you should always err on the side of caution and start small, building up. You should never apply an extension that more than doubles the natural lashes size and weight.

Some signs that you are using extensions that are too thick will include difficulty or prolonged time with the adhesive setting while you are applying the extensions. This is because a larger extension will pick up more glue, and with less surface area on the natural lash for it to spread to, the longer time it will take to cure. As a result, the application process takes longer, is harder to do, and it is more likely that you will have multiple lashes stuck together. With that said, lashes that stick together despite isolation during the application, is another sign that the extensions you are choosing may be too wide. If the extensions weigh down the natural lash, or twist or break off between fill appointments, you are applying lashes that are too large or heavy for the client's natural lash. Remember that applying lashes that are too large may cause permanent damage to your clients' lash follicles. This must be avoided at all costs.

With all that in mind, here are a few starter tips:

- 0.15mm lashes are most often a safe size to start with, especially if you choose a conservative length (which you should do to start).
- 0.10mm – 0.12mm lashes are more suitable for people with thinner and weaker lashes.
- 0.18 – 0.20mm lashes may be used only on people with strong enough lashes to support them.
- Extensions larger than 0.20mm width are too thick, will weigh too much and will not give you quality results.
- For a natural look, extend the natural lash length by 2-3mm.
- For a more dramatic look, extend the natural lash length by 3-4mm.

- If you are using flat lashes, you may be able to apply thicker, longer lashes without adding too much weight.
- Err on the side of caution and then build up size from there.

Classic Lash Selection

For a classic eyelash extension application the goal is to create a full, more voluptuous natural look to your client's eyes. This set of lashes may initially take you up to 3 hours to complete. As you become more skilled it is possible to complete a full classic set in 1.5 to 2 hours. Your client's natural lashes limit you as to what you can achieve. You should not apply a lash extension that is too heavy or too long for the natural lash to support. The rule of thumb when selecting eyelash extensions is to never more than double the weight of a natural lash. It should be your goal to attach an eyelash extension to every natural eyelash. Some people have large numbers of natural eyelashes making that impossible. And some eyelash extension artists prefer to offer a quicker service and bond extensions only to every 3rd or 4th natural lash regardless. The number of natural lashes that you attach an extension to will modify the fullness of your finished extensions. And if you choose to attach lashes sparingly, your clients will need to return for fill appointments more often. This will end up costing them more money in the long run.

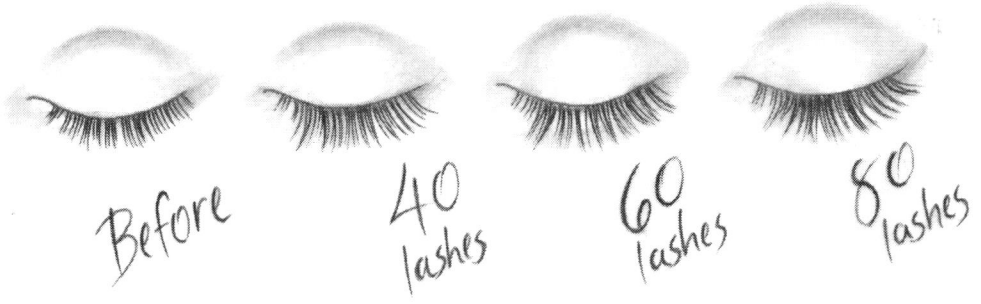

Before   40 lashes   60 lashes   80 lashes

For a classic set of extensions, one extension will be attached to one natural eyelash. The lash curl selected will most often be a J, B, or C curl, depending on the client's natural eye shape and desired outcome. The width of the lash selected for a classic set of extensions is most commonly a 0.15mm. Extensions with 0.15mm width tend to be the same as or slightly thicker than natural lashes. The increased thickness creates the look and feel of volume, even with no makeup applied.

For a more dramatic look, if the client's natural lashes are sturdy enough to manage a thicker lash, you may choose to select a 0.18 - 0.20mm width. These will have a fancier, more artificial look and feel to them when the set is completed. They are also harder to apply with isolation. The larger lashes require more glue, which increases your chances of sticking multiple lashes together. Use larger lash widths only with extreme care.

You may also wish to apply a classic set of extensions using a thinner width of 0.10mm or 0.12mm. These will offer a softer, more natural finished look and may be perfect for the client who doesn't want the look of drama! Thinner, lighter lashes are less likely to have a fake feel for the client. The below image shows a complete classic set of 0.10 brown lashes applied for a client who didn't want people to know she had extensions at all.

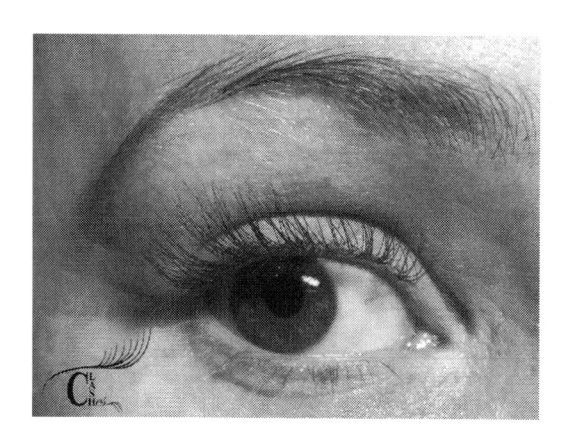

Lash Mapping

There is room for a lot of creativity in eyelash extension selection. You can simply enhance the natural look, or you can make smaller eyes look bigger with a dramatic doll-eyed style application. You can create the look of playfulness, with camel-styled eyelashes, or even give your client a sleepy, sultry, sassy cat-eyed look. With time and practice, you'll soon learn what lashes work best to achieve which looks.

Lash mapping is the term given to selecting and mapping the lashes you will use, to create a specific lash look. Most often used when volume lashing, eyelash extension artists will either draw lines on the under eye pad, or purchase pads with pre-drawn lines, that create up to 8 or 9 different sections, as shown in the following image.

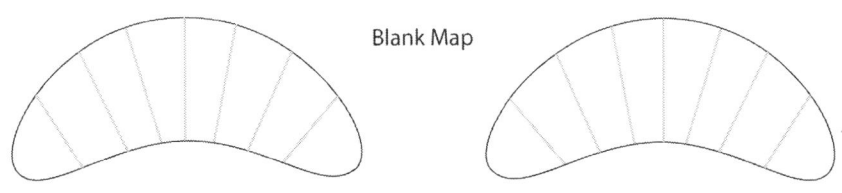

Blank Map

The length, size and curl of the extension to be used may be written in each section of the pad, mapping out the extensions chosen for the desired look. This serves as a reminder or a map to follow while you work and the maps can be shared with other artists so they can achieve a similar look in their work. The following table shows some varying looks that can be created for an eyelash extension set, and it describes the extension choices that may have created these looks.

Natural Classic
J-curl
0.15mm
Lash map: 9mm at the outside of the eye to 10mm through the middle to 8mm at the inside of the eye. This map may be written and shared as *9/10/11/11/11/11/10/9/8*.

Dramatic Doll Eyes
C or D-curl
0.15mm
Lash map: 9mm at the outside of the eye to 12mm at the middle of the eye to 9mm at the inside of the eye. This map may be written and shared as *9/10/11/12/12/11/10/9*

Camel
C or D-curl
0.15mmm
Lash map: 10mm at the outside of the eye to 8mm at the inside of the eye. This map may be written and shared as *10/11/11/11/11/10/9/8*.

Cat Eyes
C or D-curl at the outside of the eye, J-curls through the middle and inside of the eye
0.15mm
Lash map: 11mm & 12mm at the outside of the eye to 8mm at the inside of the eye. This map may be written and shared as *11/12/12/11/10/9/8*.

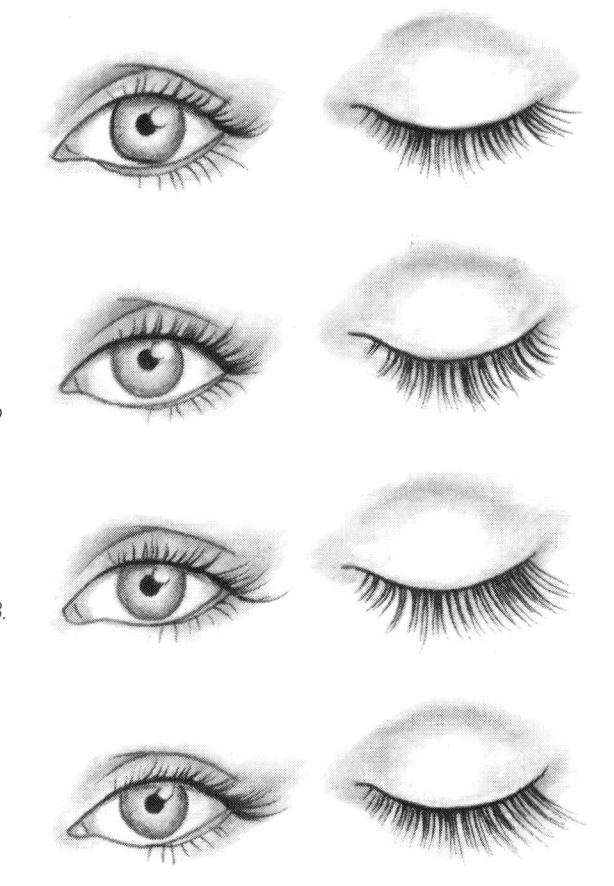

You'll notice that the lashes mapped at the very outside and inside of the eye are the smallest. Even when you're aiming to create a dramatic style, like cat eyes or camel, the very outside and inside lashes should have slightly smaller extensions attached. This is for your client's comfort. Using a couple of different lengths will maintain a natural appearance, regardless of the style you are aiming to create. Your natural eyelashes are all different lengths and your extensions should be as well.

In practice, you will aim to attach a shorter extension to a shorter natural lash, and a longer extension to a longer natural lash. A shorter natural lash still has more growing to do, and if you attach the longest extension to a shorter lash, it will result in the extension being noticeably longer compared to the others and the eventual bending or breaking of the natural eyelash as it grows. As you move from a longer group of lashes, say at the middle of the eye, to the shorter lashes on the inside of the eye, you will gradually work the shorter lashes into the larger ones so the lash length transition is smooth.

Popular Eyelash Extension Maps
The following are some of the more popular eyelash extension maps.

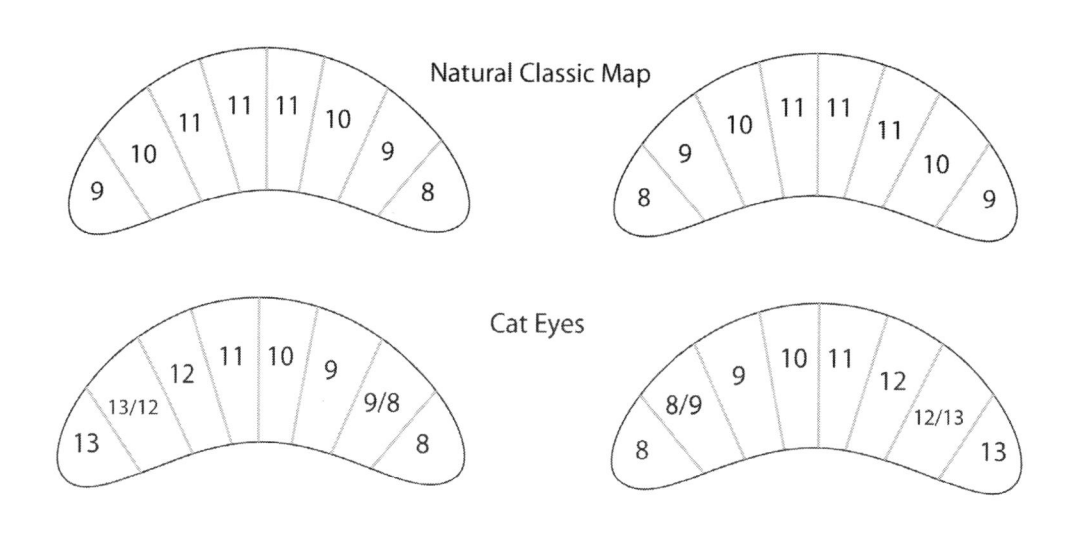

Natural Classic Map

Cat Eyes

Open/Doll Eyes

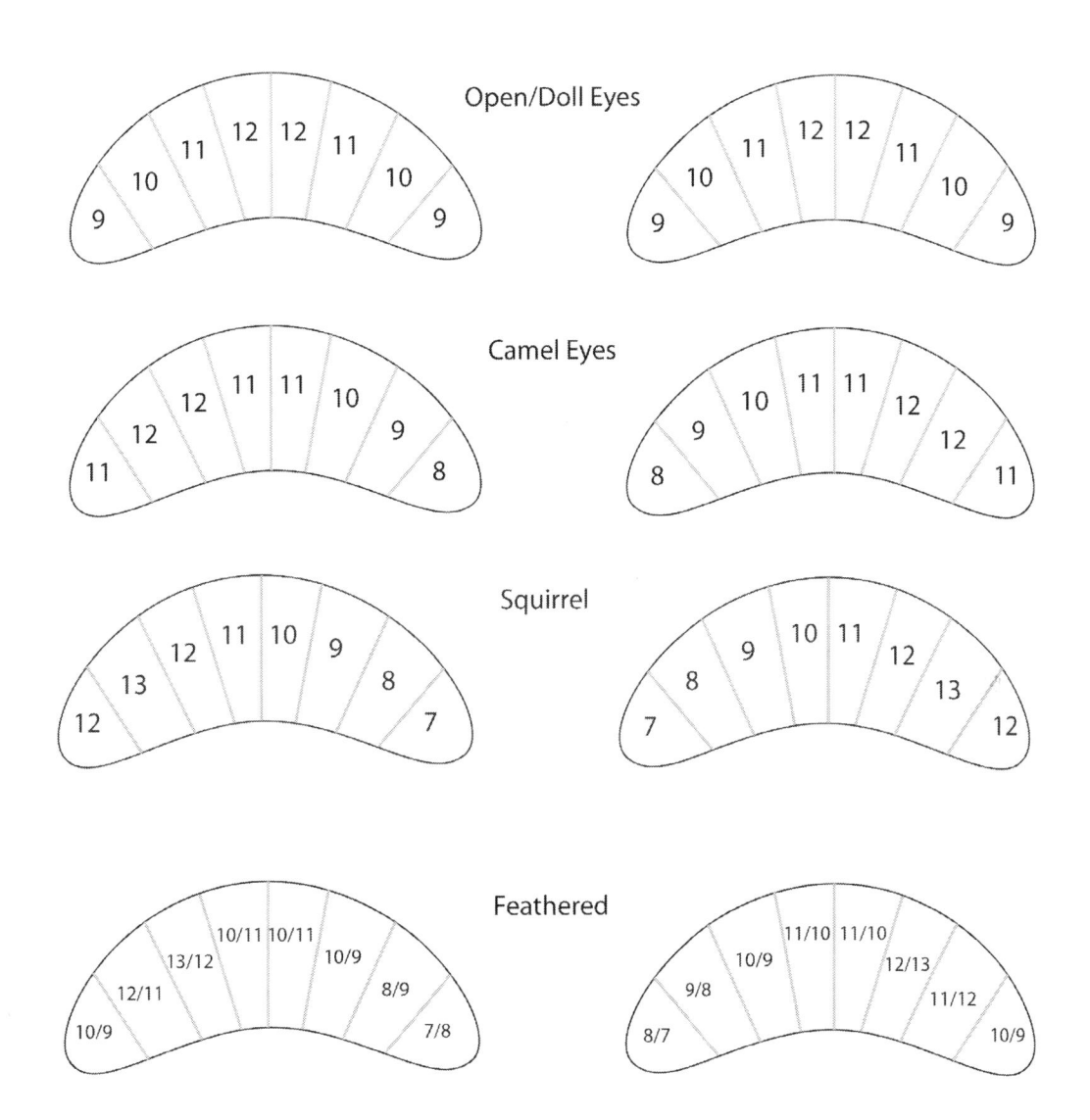

Left eye (from outer to inner): 9, 10, 11, 12, 12, 11, 10, 9
Right eye (from inner to outer): 9, 10, 11, 12, 12, 11, 10, 9

Camel Eyes

Left eye: 11, 12, 11, 11, 10, 9, 8
Right eye: 8, 9, 10, 11, 11, 12, 12, 11

Squirrel

Left eye: 12, 13, 12, 11, 10, 9, 8, 7
Right eye: 7, 8, 9, 10, 11, 12, 13, 12

Feathered

Left eye: 10/9, 12/11, 13/12, 10/11, 10/11, 10/9, 8/9, 7/8
Right eye: 8/7, 9/8, 10/9, 11/10, 11/10, 12/13, 11/12, 10/9

For a client who has shorter, thinner lashes, you may subtract 1mm or 2mm from each of these mapped lengths. For a client who has stronger, longer natural lashes you may add 1mm or 2mm to each of these mapped lengths.

Natural Eye Shapes & Choosing Lash Styles

You are limited in the eyelash style you can achieve by your clients eyelashes as well as their natural eye shape. Some lash styles will simply look better with one eye shape than it would on another other.

Round, Oval or Almond Shaped Eyes

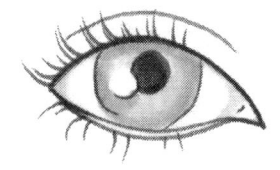

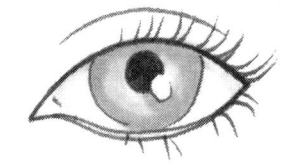

Oval shaped eyes are seen as open, bright and pointed at both sides. You'll notice the space between the lash line and the crease in the lid allows for room to see the eyelashes. Just about any eyelash extension style that takes the emphasis away from the middle and creates a cat-eye flick at the outer edge will elongate the appearance of the eye, and look chic on this eye shape. Use a B or C curl, depending on the amount of drama your client is looking to achieve. Avoid D & L curls, as they may create a startled look. Work with your client's request and the natural lash abilities to hold extension weight, and they're almost guaranteed to be thrilled!

Close Set Eyes

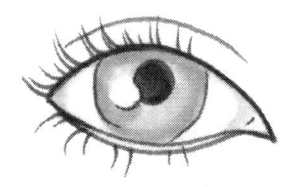

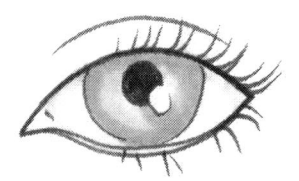

If the space between a person's eyes is less than the width of one of their eyes, that person has close set eyes. As with round or oval shaped eyes, you'll aim to elongate the look using B & C curls with the emphases on the outer corner. Do not use a doll-eye style as this will lead to a startled look.

Wide Set Eyes

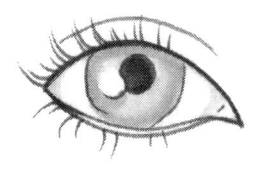

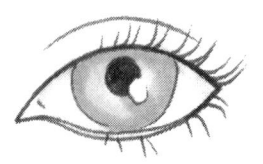

If the space between a person's eyes is larger than the width of one of their eyes, they have what's referred to as wide set eyes. You'll aim to reduce the appearance of the space between the eyes by using a doll-eyed effect with the emphasis at the center of the eye, and a deep curl like a C or D. Avoid using a cat-eyed styles, as this will only elongate the eyes further and exaggerate the appearance of wider set eyes.

Hooded Eyes

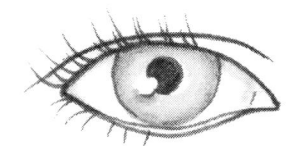

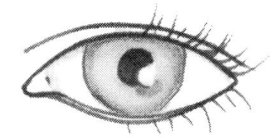

In hooded eyes, often seen in elder women, the creases of the eyelids are closer to the lash line and not as easily seen as in round eyes. Use a B curl at the outside of the eyes and L curls or longer lengthen C curls through the center, to help disguise the hood and make the eyes look larger and brighter. Avoid anything with a deep curl like D, as this may curl back and touch the lid.

Monolid

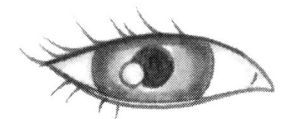

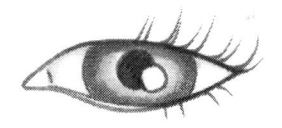

As the name suggests, monolid eyes have no eyelid crease, or the eyelid crease is so low it reaches beyond the lash line and the opening of the eye. Often seen in Asian populations, this natural shape can hide the natural eyelashes under the lid, so that it appears the eye has no lashes at all. Much like a hooded eye, use B curls on the outside of the eye to elongate the eye, and L curls through the middle may work best, to extend the lashes out beyond the reaches of the eyelid and create the appearance of more open eyes. L curls add length and drama, and are often used in this population. If L curls are not available to you, you may find longer length C curls work as well.

Deep Set Eyes

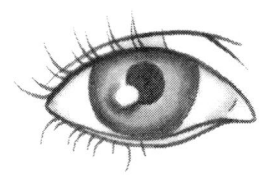

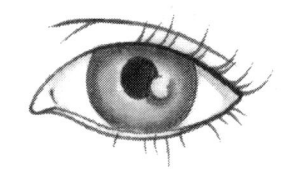

This eye shape often appears to be set deeper within the face. Longer extensions with a B or C curl, to bring the appearance of the eyes forward, are most flattering.

Down Turned Eyes

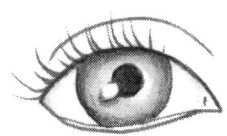

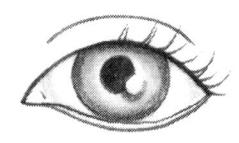

Down turned eyes, with the outer edge resting lower than the inner edge, tend to have a droopy feel to them. Your aim is to create the appearance of lifting the eyes up. While this eye shape is perfect for doll-eyed, a full classic natural style set using a deep curl like C or D will help lift these eyes right up! You will want to avoid J and B curls and a cat eye effect on this client, as these will emphasize the droopy appearance.

When selecting the extension style that will work best for your client, work with them, their natural lashes, and their requests. It may take a while for you to recognize the different eye shapes, and to determine which style works best. Remember that with a classic styled set, where you follow the natural length patterns of the eyelashes and apply shorter extensions to shorter natural lashes and longer extensions to longer natural lashes, you cannot go wrong!

Apply Lower Lash Barrier
Once you've made your extension selections, wash your hands thoroughly. You are now ready to start the actual application process. The first step is to apply the lower lash barrier. Keep in mind that the client's eye shape will help determine how well your lower lash barrier fits or does not fit to the eye. Whether you are using a gel pad or sticker, the

application process is similar, and you have multiple options for the order in which you apply things.

With your client lying on their back, and you seated at the top of the table above your client's head, have your client open their eyes and look up towards the ceiling, towards you, or towards their own forehead. By looking up, they open their eyelids fully, which in most cases, makes it easier to place the barrier over the lower lashes while avoiding the upper lashes. How far up or close to you they need to look will vary, depending on their lower eyelid movement. If the under eye barrier slides up when they close their eyes, their under eyelid may be extremely animated and they may have looked too far up towards you. If you can adjust the barrier with their eyes closed so that it fits comfortably, do so. If not, you may have to try again without have them look so far up. There are some people who have lower lids that move so much upon opening and closing the eyes, it's best to try and apply the extensions with their eyes closed, or almost closed to begin with. You do this by gently pulling up the upper lid to apply the pad. This is an advanced technique that I do not recommend you attempt without proper hands-on instruction.

If your client has almond shaped eyes, where the gel pad or sticker you are using perfectly fits over the lower lash line, you may place your sticker or gel pad directly over the lower lashes, tacking them down. Be sure to separate the lower lashes from the upper lashes so that you are not tacking down any of the upper lashes with the lower, especially at the outside corner of the eye where the upper and lower lashes tend to mingle. Using micropore tape, you may tack down any of the lower lashes that were not caught by the gel pad or sticker.

For most other eye shapes, you will do this process in reverse. Tack the lower eyelashes down with micropore tape first, and then apply the gel or sticker pads over the tape. This allows for the maximum amount of lower lash coverage and is convenient when the lower lashes are thick and firm and do not want to tack down under a gel pad or eye sticker alone, or when the client has a natural concavity below the eye that prevents the pad from sticking. This method helps prevent the bruising of the eyeball in people with really round eyes, and by taping below the gel pad or sticker, it tends to do a better job of keeping the lower lashes tacked down during the application process.

The tape will pull on the lower lashes during removal more than the gel pad will, but neither gel pad nor medical tape should pluck out the lashes. If you feel your micropore tape is too tacky, you may de-tack it first by sticking and then pulling it off of the back of your clean hand a few times, before placing it. Alternatively, you may apply a very thin layer of unscented oil-free cream created for use around the eye, to the area under the eye before tacking the lashes down. When taping the lashes down first, you may use four pieces of tape, that crisscross below the eye. This ensures that even if the gel pads or stickers do not fit to each side of the eye exactly the lower lashes will still all be covered. Gel pads are one uniform size that varies only between brands. Eye shapes are not!

Step 1:

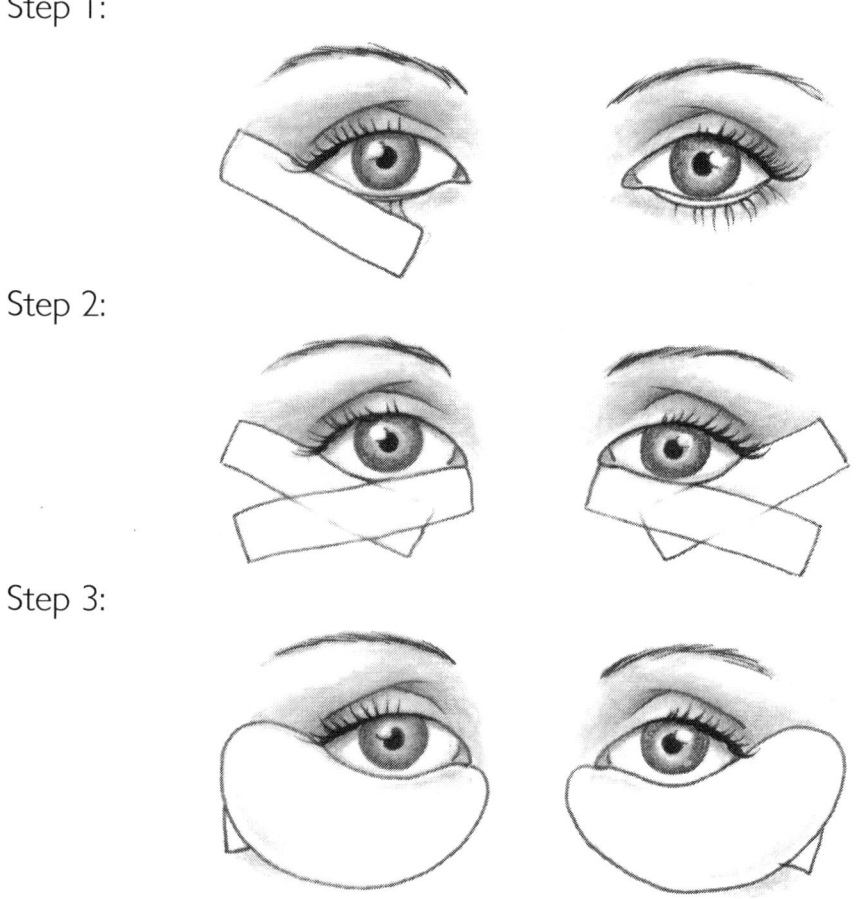

Step 2:

Step 3:

Once you've applied the under eye barrier, have your client close their eyes and confirm that they are comfortable. This is important because any discomfort may cause your client's eyes to water during the application process. If they are not comfortable, make any adjustments necessary to the barrier and check again. Once the barrier is comfortably in place, ask your client to keep their eyes closed for the remainder of the application process.

Cleanse & Prime Natural Lashes

Using cotton swabs, or a disposable makeup brush, and a gentle eyelash cleanser, clean the eyelashes so that no makeup, oil or other grit remains. By turning their head to the side of the eye that you are working on, and placing a paper towel below that same side of the face, you may rinse the cleanser off using a distilled water or saline solution. You may prefer to ask your clients to wash any makeup off their face before their appointment to reduce the amount of time you spend cleansing and priming the lashes. Often there will still be makeup residue left on the eyelashes after they have cleaned them, and you may have to cleanse them yourself anyway. Once the lashes are clean, dry them with your eyelash puffer or dryer.

Apply the eyelash primer using a micro brush being careful not let the primer drip onto the client's eyelid or into the eye. Remember the contents of the primer include alcohol. Once the primer has been applied, use a disposable eyelash wand to evenly brush the primer through all of the lashes. Dry with your eyelash puffer, fan or dryer if necessary.

Do not skip priming. Failing to prime the eyelashes will result in a weak bond between the eyelash extension and the natural eyelash. Your extensions will fall off prematurely. There are some arguments that alcohol-based primers dry out the natural lashes. This would only be the case if the lashes were dry to start with, and the exposure to alcohol was repeated consistently. The natural eyelash cycle results in the natural loss of lashes, long before the priming of the lashes can cause any damage. The benefits of better retention and a smoother application base outweigh the potential cons.

If at any time throughout the application process from here forward, your client feels product or fumes seep into their eyes, you may mist with water or fan with a puffer until relief is achieved. If misting and fanning do not quickly achieve relief, administer first aid.

Determine Application Pattern & Isolate Natural Eyelash

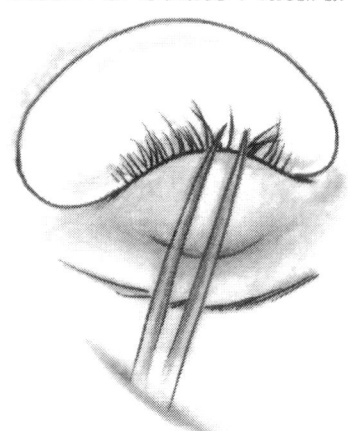

Eyelash extensions are usually applied either by following a 3-step pattern of a middle lash first, an outside lash second, then an inside lash last, repeated until all the eyelash extensions are attached, or they are applied by attaching an extension to the outer most lashes first and working towards the inner eyelashes one-by-one. My personal preference is working from outer to the inner lashes as I find lash isolation is easier this way and I'm certain to attach an extension to as many natural eyelashes as possible, without missing any. Eventually, pattern selection will come naturally to you. No matter which pattern you prefer, you must master the art of isolating one natural eyelash using the isolation tweezers and you should work back and forth from eye-to-eye. This is especially important when you are new, and are getting used to isolating lashes while the glue sets. Advanced lashes may find it's quicker completely lash one eye and then move on to the next.

The straight tweezers are held in your non-dominant hand (the left hand for most people), and are used to separate the natural lashes until one lash is standing alone in isolation, without any other natural or artificial eyelash attached to it or near to it. This is crucial for making sure that you do not attach one extension to multiple natural lashes.

Apply Extensions

When applying the eyelash extensions, you will apply an artificial eyelash, or a few extensions, to one eye and then let it, or them, set while you apply an extension, or a few, to the other eye, working back and forth between both eyes. Applying lashes in this manner allows for the newly applied extensions to dry and set with minimal clumping together in the surrounding eyelashes.

Once you have an eyelash isolated, you will use your curved-nosed tweezers, held in your dominant hand, to pick up the artificial lash you wish to attach to the isolated natural lash. Dip the artificial eyelash just a millimeter or two into the glue so that one or two tiny drops of glue can be seen on the base of the extension. The goal is to use the least amount of glue possible to create the strongest possible bond between the extension and the natural eyelash.

You need to maintain fresh glue throughout the application process. As time progresses you will notice that the glue becomes tacky, stringy and thick. Remember that thicker glue will take longer to set and will increase the chances of multiple lashes being stuck together. Use fresh glue drops as required throughout the application process.

When applying the extension to the lash you must secure the very base of the extension to the natural eyelash near its base, so that the base of the extension lays flat against the natural lash. The tips of the extension and the natural lash may not be secured together, especially if you are applying a high-curl extension to a straight lash. If you are attempting to attach an extension to naturally curly lash, you may find it's easiest to attach the extension to the side of the natural lash, rather than on top.

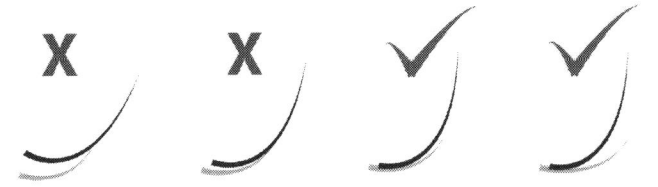

Some eyelash extension artists will encourage sweeping the extension over the natural eyelash a few times, to coat it with glue, before dropping the extension into place to set. While, when using a black colored eyelash extension glue, this can help you see light colored or very fine natural lashes, and it may increase the surface area of the bond, it is not essential to the longevity of the extensions and may even prolong the time it takes for the adhesive to set and/or encourage multiple lashes to stick together, especially if you use too much adhesive to do this. I do not recommend doing this.

The more adhesive on the lash extension when you attach it to the natural lash, the longer it will take to set and dry, and the more likely it will be that multiple natural eyelashes get stuck to the same extension. More adhesive creates more weight, and the more weight that is added to the individual lash, the more stress is placed on the natural eyelash. This can lead to discomfort for the client and for the extensions to eventually twist, break and fall out. If multiple lashes are glued together, and not separated, it will lead to the premature plucking of natural lashes due to the different rates at which each eyelash grows. Recall that an eyelash plucked out prematurely may take up to eight weeks to grow back and that repeated plucking of eyelashes may lead to permanent damage of the eyelash follicles resulting in no eyelash growth at all.

If you have too much adhesive on the eyelash extension, you can gently wipe excess amounts off on the under-eye barrier. Having too little glue will result in an inefficient bond, and extensions that do not last. Getting just the right amount necessary is learned through practice.

Once you have an appropriate amount of glue on the extension, place the base of the eyelash extension on the isolated natural lash, 0.5-1mm away from the eyelid. Do not touch or attach the eyelash extension to the eyelid itself. A properly applied extension, in the proper environment will set in 3-6 seconds. If the extension fails to attach with the first attempt, you may try again with the same lash, however, you should not dip the same extension in glue multiple times over as it may lead to too much glue being applied and a weaker, less consistent bond. It's better to discard an extension than to reuse an extension that has failed.
As you are learning to lash, always point the sharp tips of the curved tweezers away from your client's face, towards their feet or the side of the table. The long base of the tweezers' mouth is maintained in a

position that is parallel to the face so that if the tweezers slip out of your hand, it is not the point that falls into your client's eyes. This grip is also necessary for building volume fans, as we'll discuss later.

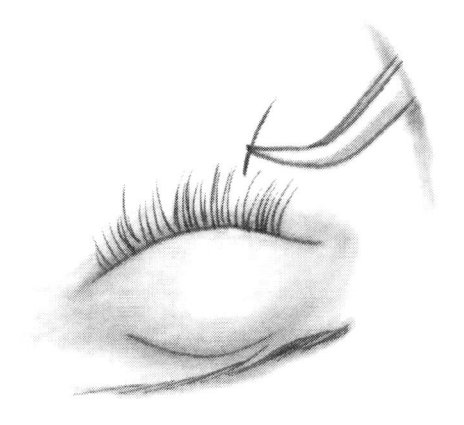

Repeat the process of isolating a natural lash, dipping the artificial eyelash extension in glue, and attaching it to the isolated lash, moving from eye to eye until all the eyelash extensions have been applied.

During this application process, especially when you are new to applying extensions, you may find that bits of glue adhere lash extensions to your tweezers, making the extensions reluctant to fall off and difficult to place on your client's natural lash. The easiest and most efficient way to clean glue from your tweezers during application is to gently file the glue off with a fine nail file. You may not want to do this with extremely pricey tweezers. Adhesive can be cleaned from expensive tweezers using acetone, but the tweezers must then be properly rinsed with water before using them on your client's lashes again.

Inspection & Lash Separation

Once all the extensions have been applied, fan the eyelashes with your puffer or an eyelash fan for 30-60 seconds each eye. This helps any remaining glue to dry and will dissipate any glue fumes away from the eye. Use your tweezers to inspect each and every individual lash by separating them one-by-one. Make sure each lash can be isolated and is not stuck to the protective under-eye barrier below or to multiple lashes beside it. Using the tweezers, gently lift any lashes that are stuck to the lower lash barrier so that they can move independently. If you find two or more lashes stuck together gently peel the lashes apart. If absolutely necessary you may use your adhesive remover or cosmetic scissors to separate lashes that are stuck to one another. We will cover how to remove individual extensions with adhesive removers in a later chapter.

Only cut lashes with extreme caution, cutting just one single lash at a time. Do not cut multiple lashes side-by-side, or an entire clump of multiple lashes that are stuck together. Eyelashes, both natural and artificial, have tapered ends. Cutting them will leave a very unappealing, blunt-edged look. While it is best to avoid cutting the lashes all together, it is more important that no two lashes are left stuck together. Practice, patience, and technique are imperative here.

Final Comb Through, Setting & Finishing Up

Once you've inspected the lashes to ensure that they all move independently of each other, comb through the eyelashes with the disposable eyelash wand. Make sure you've removed all adhesives from the area of your client's face. If you are in a dry climate, you may need to mist the eyelashes with distilled water prior to fanning, in order to help the glue fully set. While this is not a necessary step in extremely humid environments, it helps to ensure that any remaining glue sets immediately. Then fan and brush the lashes again for up to 60 seconds on each eye to dissipate any remaining fumes and make the lashes look finished.

Some eyelash extension artists will also coat the dry, finished extensions with a mascara-like product known as an eyelash extension sealant. This is not a necessary step, but one of preference. I do not use, nor recommend, the use of sealants for my clients. Eyelash extensions are meant to be low maintenance!

Gently remove the lower lash barriers and ask your client to slowly open their eyes. If they feel any pulling, or discomfort in opening their eyes, you may have missed separating an eyelash bonded to the lower lid, or a lower eyelash that has stuck itself to an upper extensions. Inspect and gently correct. Once corrected, the eyelash extension application is complete. Give your client a mirror so they may see their new eyelashes.

Classic Extension Application Step-by-Step
1. Set up your workstation before your client arrives.
2. Consult with your client, have them fill out any necessary forms, and make lash extension selection.
3. If your client arrives wearing heavy make up, ask them to wash their face before you begin.
4. Instruct your client how to position themselves on the table and wash your hands while the client makes himself or herself comfortable.
5. Assist the client in positioning their head so that it is both comfortable and in a position where you can work without the eyelashes sticking to the lower pad.
6. Apply lower lash barriers.
7. Cleanse and prime the upper eyelashes.
8. Put a drop of glue on your glue ring, jade stone or other glue holder. Shake the bottle vigorously first!
9. Isolate the client's natural lash and apply extensions, working in a pattern of preference, being sure to move back and forth from eye to eye.
10. Remember to inspect, separate, brush and fan the lashes as you work, once for approximately every 10-15 lashes applied to each eye.
11. When all lashes have been applied, inspect and separate. Make sure no upper lashes are stuck to the lower lash pad or to other lashes.
12. Seal your work by misting the finished job with water.
13. Fan dry and brush the lashes.
14. Gently remove the under eye pads.
15. Give your client their after care instruction sheet.
16. Take payment and book your client's next fill appointment.
17. A full classic application should take less than 3 hours to complete.

Fill Appointment Applications

For an eyelash extension fill appointment, you will follow similar steps as in the original application process, only you will start with more preparation. After cleansing the eyelashes, you will inspect and separate the lashes as you normally do at the end of the eyelash extension application appointment. Depending on the aftercare regime that your client adheres to, the length of time between appointments, and the state of your client's lashes when they come in, you may spend some time preparing the old extensions in order to apply new fill extensions. You may have to remove some of the old extensions due to congealed glue, or an extension deformity (like the loss of curl) before you can successfully apply new ones. Once the lashes are prepared and separated, you will follow the regular application steps as previously covered. New eyelash extensions are applied to new-growth natural lashes and existing natural lashes where the old extensions have fallen off.

Fill Appointment Step-by-Step

1. Set up your workstation before your client arrives.
2. Consult with your client, have them fill out any necessary forms, and make lash extension selection.
3. If your client arrives wearing heavy make up, ask them to wash their face before you begin.
4. Instruct your client how to position themselves on the table and wash your hands while the client makes himself or herself comfortable.
5. Assist the client in positioning their head so that it is both comfortable and in a position where you can work without the eyelashes sticking to the lower pad.
6. Apply lower lash barriers.
7. Cleanse and prime the upper eyelashes, removing any old extensions as necessary.
8. Put a drop of glue on your glue ring, jade stone or other glue holder. Shake the bottle vigorously first!
9. Isolate new, natural lashes and apply extensions
10. Remember to inspect, separate, brush and fan the lashes as you work, once for approximately every 10-15 lashes applied to each eye.
11. When all lashes have been applied, inspect and separate. Make sure no upper lashes are stuck to the lower lash pad or to other lashes.
12. Seal your work by misting the finished job with water.
13. Fan dry and brush the lashes.
14. Gently remove the under eye pads.
15. Give your client their after care instruction sheet.

16. Take payment and book your client's next fill appointment.

Application Tips & Tricks

When applying eyelash extensions, the more tricks you have to make your job easier, the better the end results will be. The following tips and tricks have made my application process smoother and my results more consistent.

Hooded Eyelids & Lash Angles

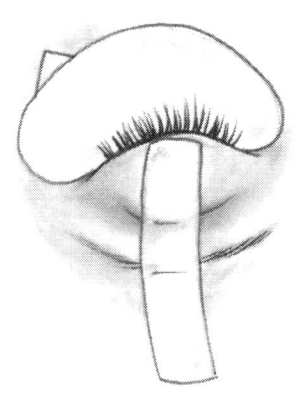

If your client's natural anatomy is hooded upper eyelids, you may find that the eyelid interferes with your access to the eyelashes. A simple fix for this is to lift the eyelids while you work, using a small piece of micropore tape. Tacking one end of the tape to the eyelid, gently pull the lid up, to reduce the eyelid slack, being careful not to pull open the eye. Tack the other end of the tape just above the eyebrow. Be sure to apply a thin layer of petroleum jelly over the eyebrows before taping, to ensure that the tape does not pull out any of the eyebrow hair when removed.

This taping method may also be used to angle the natural lashes for clients with extremely straight natural eyelashes or to access condensed-growing inner eyelashes. Without manipulating the lashes with tape as described, really straight natural lashes may have the tendency to rest on the lower lash barrier, increasing the likelihood for the extensions to stick to the lower lid barrier during the application.

By angling the upper portion of the tape more towards the outer eyebrow, or even taping from the mid-upper eyelid to the outside of the eye with gentle traction, avoiding the eyebrow all together, you can pull the lid and the lash line towards the outside of the eye, to make the inner eyelashes near the inner eye more spacious and easily accessible.

Taping Up

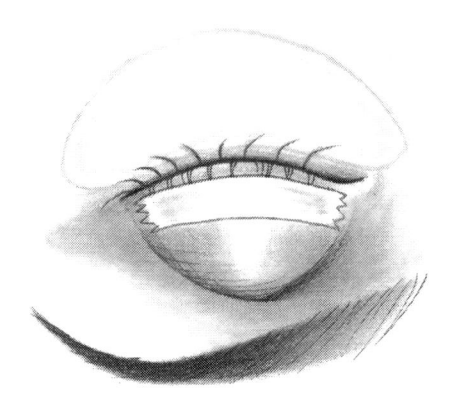

Whether you're doing a fill application or a full application using a patterned approach, getting at the lowest layer of new growth lashes can be a challenge. To access these lashes you may use a disposable eyelash wand to hold the longer, higher lashes out of your way while you work, or you may use a tack-reduced piece of tape to hold the longer lashes back, in a method referred to as taping up. To tape up lashes, first reduce the tape tack by sticking the tape to the back of your clean hand, and then removing it. Do this a couple of times until the tape is not so tacky that it will tug on the eyelashes as you remove it. Apply the tape to the bottom-side of the very tips of the eyelash extensions, pulling them up and away from the lower layer of lashes to give you access. Be sure not to pull open your client's eye!

Increasing Glue Longevity
To increase the life of your lash glue, store it in the fridge between appointments. Be sure to bring it out of the fridge a few hours before use, so that it can return to its proper consistency at room temperature. There is some debate as to whether or not condensation will develop inside the glue bottle, causing the pre-mature spoiling of the glue. Chemically, this would only occur if your environment was very humid

and you left the lid off the glue for long periods of time so that new, wet air could make its way into the glue. Some eyelash extensions artists will even store their glue in an airtight container, which also contains a silica package to ensure a moisture-free environment, prior to placing it in the fridge.

Like any super glue, you may find it difficult to keep the cap from sticking to the dispenser part of the bottle, or you may find that the thin dispenser tube glues itself closed. You can prevent this from happening by discarding the cap and using a thumbtack instead, pressed into the dispenser tube, to seal the bottle tightly between uses. After shaking your glue before use, twist the thumbtack in a clockwise, or counter-clockwise motion, to release the pin, before removing it. Take the pin out only to dispense your glue drop before use and then promptly seal the bottle again to minimize the contents exposure to air.

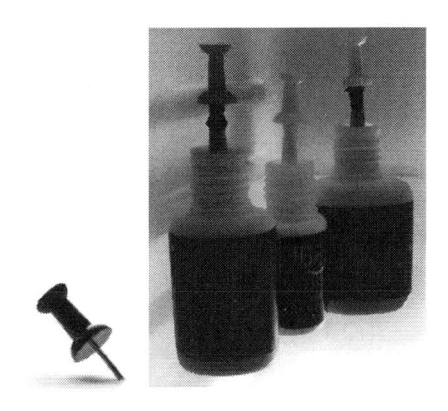

Glue Holder Clean Up

When using a glue ring, a jade stone, or some other glue holder, the best way to clean up the leftover glue is to submerge your glue holder in 100% pure acetone. In my practice, I have a small jar that is filled with acetone at my workstation. As soon as I am done with my glue ring, I place it in the acetone bath and tightly screw on the lid. Once every couple of days fish all the rings out and rinse them thoroughly with warm water. By bathing the glue holders in acetone, they are cleaned of remaining eyelash glue and are disinfected between uses.

Mid-Application Breaks

If for any reason your client needs to open their eyes during the application process, it is possible to do so. Ask them to advise you in advance. Do a quick inspection to make sure no lashes are stuck to the lower lash barrier, and correct any you may find. Remove your tweezers and your working glue from the area of the client's face. Fan the eyelashes for 60 seconds to dissipate any fumes. The client should be able to open their eyes without any discomfort. There is no need to remove the under-eye lash barrier for short breaks.

Chapter Summary Points

- The information contained in this book is not meant to replace hands-on learning.
- Your client's natural eyelashes limit eyelash extension selection and style options you have.
- The eyelash extension application process always starts with properly cleaned and sterilized hands and tools.
- Tips and tricks can make your job easier!

Definitions

Micropore tape	a paper tape used to dress wounds and secure medical tubing, that allows skin to breathe

12. Volume & Russian Volume Application

All volume eyelash extensions are created using fanned 0.10mm or smaller width extensions. The smaller extension width ensures that a low weight fan of multiple lashes can be applied to a single, isolated natural lash. This is necessary for the extension longevity and natural eyelash health. We've already discussed how too much weight on a natural lash can lead to bending or the premature falling off of the eyelash extension. You should never build or apply volume extensions using a lash extension that is larger than 0.10mm.

The difference between regular volume lashes and Russian volume lashes is whether or not the eyelash extension artists create the fans themselves, attaches and fans the lashes individually one-by-one on the natural lash, or uses a pre-made fan. There is some talk of American Volume and Hollywood Volume. American Volume is a set built with Russian Volume fans made with multiple length extensions. What's being referred to as Hollywood Volume, is simply extremely long Russian Volume fans.

Pre-made volume fans are created with anywhere from 2 to 20, 0.07mm or smaller single eyelash extensions all tacked together at the base. They are referred to as 2D through 20D extensions. The D describes each individual extension; the number before it describes how many extensions are tacked together into one fan. For professional use, fans will be adhered together into a fine point at the base, so that it can be attached to a single isolated natural eyelash. Fans are also created and sold for personal use. Personal use fans are tied in a knot instead of glued together at the base and are referred to as 'clusters'. Clusters cannot be applied to an isolated natural lash. Cluster fans are attached to the eyelid using glue that is specifically formulated for use on skin. They should never be applied using professional eyelash extension glue.

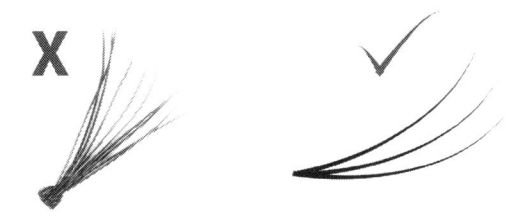

Pre-made 7D or higher fans are too heavy and too large at the base to attach to the average individual isolated eyelash. These should also never be applied using professional eyelash extension glue.

Using pre-made fans is the quickest way to achieve volume. However, quality and longevity of the eyelash extensions are compromised, dependent on the quality of the pre-made fan, and the amount of glue that is adhered to the base of the fan. The artist must be extremely careful when applying these fans, so that they are attached only to one isolated natural lash. Pre-made fans will often have a large portion of the base stuck together rather than coming together into a fine point. This results in an artificial feel and more glue being necessary to attach the fan to the individual lash, which increases the over all weight of the extension. And pre-made fans cannot hug the natural lash the way Russian volume fans can. We will look at a diagram of Russian Volume extensions hugging the natural lash a bit later.

Volume can also be achieved by applying multiple classic sets in layers, using 0.10mm or smaller extensions. The larger the lash width, the less total number of extensions can be applied to the natural lash. With a 0.10 width lash, you should not apply more than 2 extensions to the average lash natural lash, and you should only do so if the client's natural lash can handle the weight of the 2 extensions. With 0.05 width extensions you may be able to create a fan of 5 or 6 extensions per lash. Even smaller extensions, such as 0.03mm, are available, and are used for mega volume applications. Never use 0.15mm or larger width lashes to create volume sets.

With layering single extensions, the first set of lashes is applied as you normally would for a classic extension set. A second and third set can be applied on top of the first, with the second and third extensions angled out to the sides forming a fan on each individual natural eyelash. Because this method requires that each individual extension must be dipped into glue on its own, and the extensions will not hug the natural lash the way a proper Russian volume extension will, it will accumulate more weight than other methods for creating volume. For this reason, it is not recommended that you create volume in this manner using more than 3 layers. Creating volume in this manner is extremely time consuming but may be most beneficial if only used sparingly, to help fill any gaps that appear in your client's natural eyelashes.

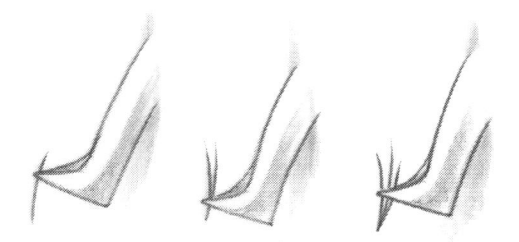

Olga Dobronravova, a Russian eyelash extension artist, first adopted the technique of creating the volume fan out of single extensions before dipping the fan in glue, thus the term **Russian Volume**. Specialty tweezers that have a mouth with maximum congruency, and that can secure and manipulate multiple lashes at the same time, are used. Multiple lashes are gently pulled from the adhesive strip of extensions and are manipulated into a fan. The base of the fanned individual lashes is then dipped into glue and the lash extensions are immediately attached to an isolated natural eyelash as a group. This technique, while requiring the most amount of practice to achieve, and taking the most amount of time to complete, is the most effective way of creating quality volume eyelash extensions with the greatest longevity.

Understanding Volume Weight

When building volume fans, one might assume that two 0.10 width lash extensions would weigh the same as a single 0.20 width lash extension. This is not the case.

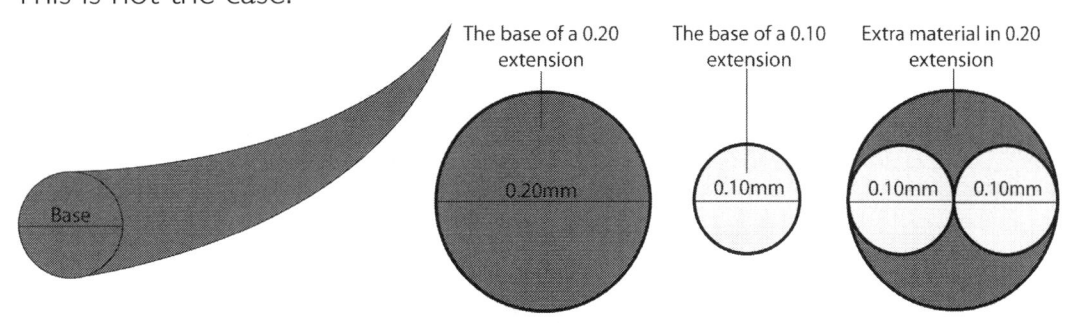

As you can see in the previous diagram, a 0.10 width lash is not exactly half the size or weight of a 0.20 width lash extension. This illustrates why it is possible to build fans with multiple single extensions of smaller widths, and why larger extension widths should be avoided when creating fans. The approximate weights of various width, 12mm long eyelash extensions are outlined in the below table.

Lash Width	Weight in Grams
.05	.0005
.07	.0006
.10	.00010
.12	.00013
.15	.00015
.20	.00030

The weight of the volume fan you can apply will ultimately depend on your client's natural eyelashes. If your client has very fine, weak natural lashes, you will choose a smaller, lighter fan. If your client has very strong lashes, you may choose to apply a fuller, heavier fan. The chart below shows how many extensions, and of which extension width, you can safely apply, depending on your clients natural lash width.

Natural Lash Width	No. Of Lashes in Fan
0.20	4 x 0.10 8 x 0.07 16 x 0.05
0.18	3 x 0.10 6 x 0.07 13 x 0.05
0.15	2 x 0.10 4 x 0.07 9 x 0.05
0.10	2 x 0.07 4 x 0.05

With time and experience you will get a feel for what works and what doesn't work. As you are learning, remember to always err on the side of caution, and work light. If your fans are twisting, bending or breaking off with growth, this is a good sign that you are applying extensions that are too heavy. A heavy extension can be uncomfortable and may ultimately cause permanent damage to your client's natural eyelashes.

Understanding Russian Volume Fan Bonding

Volume extensions will often seem to have less staying power than classic extensions. This is not always the case, but rather may seem so because with every fan that's lost, the client will lose multiple extensions. This is always true with pre-built fans, and will occur with inadequately applied Russian Fans that do not hug the natural lash, and even with the loss of the natural eyelash at the end of its growth cycle. This leads to the appearance of a gap in the lashes. Russian Volume fans should actually have a more solid bond than classic or pre-built fanned extensions. The following diagram illustrates how Russian Volume fans, when built and applied to the natural lash correctly, will hug the natural lash, causing a stronger adhesive bond than classic extensions, or even pre-built fans.

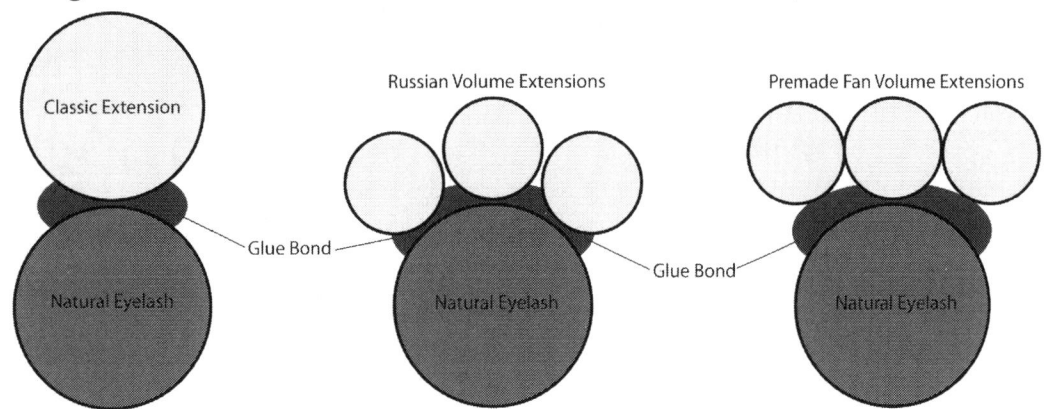

The amount of congruency between the natural lash and the extensions is increased with the addition of smaller extensions in the form of a Russian Volume fan that properly hugs the natural eyelash. Pre-built fans will not offer the same congruency as they are built so that their ends taper into a fine point, and they are applied as if they were classic single eyelash extensions. When applied correctly however, the difference in staying power between the two may be negligible.

Building Volume Fans

There are a number of different methods to create Russian Volume fans, and new techniques are emerging all the time. No matter what method you use to create volume, it will take time and practice to perfect and implement. The appointment length increases, as volume lashes tend to require more maintenance and more frequent fills than classic eyelashes. The following instructions are for information purposes only and do not serve to replace proper hands on Russian Volume fan building training. Depending on your trainer, each of the following methods may be referred to by a different name.

Building Volume Fans Method 1

1. A small bunch (3-6) of 0.05-0.07mm lashes are pulled from the adhesive strip.
2. The plucked bunch is placed lightly back onto the adhesive away from the original strip of lashes.
3. The bases of the extensions are manipulated with the closed head of the tweezers until they fan out.
4. The volume tweezers are used to pick up all of the fanned lashes simultaneously by gripping gently above the curve, being careful not to separate the bases from a fine point.
5. The bases are dipped into glue.
6. The fan is immediately attached to a single isolated natural eyelash.

Building Volume Fans Method 2

1. A small bunch (3-6) of 0.05-0.07mm lashes are pulled just 50%-70% from the grip of the adhesive strip.
2. Using the tweezers, the bases of the eyelashes are manipulated on the adhesive strip so that the tips form into a fan.
3. The volume tweezers are used to pick up all of the fanned lashes simultaneously by gripping gently above the curve, being careful not to separate the bases from a fine point.
4. The bases are dipped into glue.
5. The fan is immediately attached to a single isolated natural eyelash.

Building Volume Fans Method 3

1. A small bunch (3-6) of 0.05-0.07mm lashes are pulled just 50%-70% from the grip of the adhesive strip.
2. The tweezers are repositioned to just above the curve of the extension and the tweezers used to shimmy the extensions near the tips, to separate them into a fan.

3. The volume tweezers are used to pick up all of the fanned lashes simultaneously by gripping gently above the curve, being careful not to separate the bases from a fine point.
4. The bases are dipped into glue.
5. The fan is immediately attached to a single isolated natural eyelash.

Building Volume Fans Method 4
1. A small bunch (3-6) of 0.05-0.07mm lashes are pulled just 50%-70% from the grip of the adhesive strip.
2. The tweezers used to pull the furthest single extension to the right to create space between it and the remaining strip of extensions.
3. The lash immediately to the left of the extension that was initially pulled away is then pulled to the right as well, towards the first pulled extension, in a similar manner.
4. This process of pulling one extension to the right at a time is repeated until a fan is formed of the desired number of lashes.
5. The volume tweezers are used to pick up all of the fanned lashes simultaneously by gripping gently above the curve, being careful not to separate the bases from a fine point.
6. The bases are dipped into glue.
7. The fan is immediately attached to a single isolated natural eyelash.

Building Volume Fans Method 5
1. A small bunch (3-6) of 0.05-0.07mm lashes are pulled from the adhesive strip.
2. The plucked bunch is placed lightly back onto a piece of double-sided adhesive or mounting tape, away from the original strip of lashes.
3. The bases are placed on the mounting tape in a way that bounces the lashes into a fan.
4. The volume tweezers are used to pick up all of the fanned lashes simultaneously by gripping gently at the curve, being careful not to separate the bases from a fine point.
5. The bases are dipped into glue.
6. The fan is immediately attached to a single isolated natural eyelash.

Practicing Russian Volume

The only way to get good at creating Russian Volume fans and placing those fans on an isolated eyelash is to start practicing. There are nuances involved in creating the fans, picking up the fans, dipping them in the right amount of glue and placing the fans on the natural lash, that are difficult to describe and can only be learned by doing. Again, this book is not meant to replace a proper hands-on training course.

You must have a good set of precision tweezers. I recommend Dumont Style 7 tweezers for building fans, and Style 5/45 for lash isolation. You cannot use straight tweezers to isolate when volume lashing as you may for classic lashing. Straight isolating tweezers will get in the way as you place your volume fan. Dumont tweezers can be purchased directly from Dumont or from a scientific tool supplier. I have linked the web address for Dumont and a Canadian supplier in the resource section of this book.

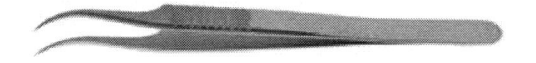

In addition to proper volume tweezers, you will need proper volume lashes with widths of 0.10 or below. I recommend starting with 0.07, C-curl as they are the most commonly used. I would recommend also buying a training mannequin and practice lashes to start. You can purchase these training assets at relatively cheap prices from my website as linked in the resource section, from Ali Express, Amazon or even eBay. Lashing is an art you can only ever improve on so practice often, no matter how good you get!

Once you have all your supplies you can start fan building practice. Try the methods above and choose the one that feels right for you. Then, using double-sided tape to secure your fans, practice building fans and then placing them on the double-sided tape. When you are comfortable with the method you've chosen graduate your practice. Start small. Practice building 2D fans, dipping them in glue, and adhering them to a makeup sponge. Make up sponges allow for quick curing of your glue, and will make obvious any imperfections in the fan base that you need to work on correcting. Work up to 5D fans. And then when you are comfortable with building fans and placing them on a sponge, graduate your practice again, so that you are practicing on your mannequin.

Chapter Summary Points

- Volume eyelash extensions can be achieved in various ways.
- Volume eyelash extensions require more maintenance than classic applications.
- All volume fans are created using fanned 0.10mm or smaller width extensions.
- Volume sets can be created using pre-built professional fans.
- Cluster fans are knotted at the bottom and are not suitable for use in professional application.
- The term Russian Volume refers to the eyelash extension artist building the fans themselves.
- The weight of two 0.10 width extensions does not equate to the weight of one 0.20 width fan.
- Russian Volume fans offer the most congruency with the natural eyelash.
- When building Russian Volume fans or using pre-made fans, you still must isolate and attach the fan to only one single natural eyelash.

Definitions

Fans	fanned eyelash extensions
Flares	see fans
Clusters	fanned extensions that are tied together in a knot and are not meant for professional use
Russian Volume	fans that are created by the eyelash extension artist at the time of extension application

13. Eyelash Extension Removal

If eyelash extensions are left unattended for long enough, the natural eyelash growth cycle will push out all of the lashes with attached extensions and replace them with new natural eyelashes. There are many reasons why a client may wish to remove their lash extensions prematurely. Complete removal may be necessary with allergic reactions, or a client's sensitivities, or simply because the client wants to take a break from having extensions and doesn't want to go through the awkward phase of having a few extensions left as the natural ones grow.

If your client suffers an allergic reaction, it is important to have the extensions removed as soon as possible. As a professional responsibility, you should always have eyelash adhesive remover available. You should also make yourself available to remove extensions in emergency situations within 24-48 hours of the original application, just in case a client reacts. Keeping this emergency removal as policy helps build your professional profile and your client confidence in your services.

In emergency removal situations, it's important that you do not panic. Your client may very well be panicking, especially if extreme symptoms present like pain or swelling of the eyelids. If you panic, too, it only increases your client's stress, and reduces their confidence in your professional abilities. The probability of an allergic reaction can be greatly reduced by performing a spot test on clients before applying a full set, as previously discussed. By making spot tests a habit, you will find yourself needing to remove only the rogue individual lash far more often than complete eyelash extension removals.

Individual Extension Removal

Individual extension removal is necessary for the rogue lash that was attached with too much glue, or was attached in a position that is not flattering, or that has come partially unattached over time. If you can remove the artificial extension by peeling it away from the natural lash without damaging or plucking out the natural lash, or hurting your client, this is the best practice as it reduces the amount of chemicals used. To peel the lashes apart, you will hold the natural lash in one set of tweezers, and the extension that is attached to it in the other set of tweezers and gently pull each eyelash towards the opposite sides of the eye and peel the lashes apart. To reduce the amount of pulling required, you may find that first squeezing the adhesive bond between tweezers will crush the glue, making the lashes easier to separate.

If you cannot peel the lashes apart, you will need to use an adhesive remover. Recall that adhesive removers are extremely powerful; therefore proceed only with extreme caution. First, make sure to apply the lower lid and lash protective barrier gel pad, or sticker, and advise your client to keep their eyes closed for the entire procedure. Using your straight tweezers, isolate the lash that needs removal from all of the other lashes. Using a micro brush, apply a small amount of adhesive remover to the base of the eyelash extension over the adhesive bond. Make sure the remover does not touch your client's eyelid. Only use enough adhesive remover to adequately cover the adhesive that bonds the extension to the natural lash. As the adhesive remover works, it creates heat and becomes more liquid. Be careful not to use so much that as it works it seeps into your client's eye. Wait a few minutes and then gently manipulate the lash extension with your curved tweezers. Within minutes, depending on the amount of adhesive to be removed, you should be able to gently peel the extension off the natural lash. Remove the extension, and any excess remover, between two micro brushes. Throw the used micro brushes away. Thoroughly wipe off any remaining adhesive remover between two new micro brushes. Again, throw the used micro brushes away. Dampen another two new micro brushes with distilled water, and gently but thoroughly cleanse the eyelash, making sure that no water seeps into your client's eyes. Repeat as necessary. Remember to properly prime the eyelash before applying a new extension.

If a lot of adhesive remover is required (for multiple individual removals or a complete extension removal), have your client seated in an upright position before you begin.

Complete Extension Removal

For complete extension removal, you must first protect the client's lower lid and lashes by applying a barrier gel pad, or sticker, and tape as you would for the application process. Have your client take a seated position and advise them to keep their eyes closed for the entire process. The seated position will ensure that as the adhesive remover works, and becomes more liquid, it seeps towards the tips of the eyelash, away from the eye, instead of towards the base of the lash and into the eye, as it would if your client were lying down as they do during the application process. Apply a thin coat of petroleum jelly to the client's upper eyelid to protect it from contact with the adhesive remover. Remove extensions from only one eye at a time, in case you need to quickly remove the adhesive remover and administer first aid.

Using a lint-free micro brush, apply only enough adhesive remover to cover the bonded area between the extensions and the natural lash of one eye. Do not allow any of the adhesive removers to touch your client's eyelid. Wait a few minutes to allow the remover to work, before carefully manipulating the extensions with your tweezers. The extensions should soon come loose from the natural lash and you should be able to gently slide them right off. Using the cotton swab, carefully wipe in a downward direction towards the tip of the eyelashes, to gently remove any remaining extensions and excess adhesive remover. Be sure not to get any of the adhesive remover on your client's cheek. Repeat as necessary until all of the eyelash extensions have been removed. Gently wipe any excess adhesive remover away using fresh cotton swabs. Dampen lint free cotton pads with filtered water or a saline solution created for use on the eyes, and thoroughly but carefully cleanse the entire area. Throw away soiled cotton pads and repeat this step as necessary, until no further adhesive remover remains. Remove the under eye barrier. Have your client lay back down on the table, with their head tilted in the direction of the eye you are working on. Place a handful of paper towels under the side of their face and rinse the eye area with distilled water or a saline solution formulated specifically for the eyes. Once completed, repeat the entire process on the other eye.

Gently dry the client's eyelashes with your eye puffer or fan. Remove the protective under-eye barriers and have your client slowly open their eyes. If the client experiences any reaction or sensation that suggests the product, or product fumes, got into their eyes, follow with first aid for product eye contact.

Complete Extension Removal Step-by-Step
1. Set up workstation before your client arrives.
2. Wash your hands while the client makes themselves comfortable on your working table.
3. Apply lower lash barrier.
4. Apply a thin coat of petroleum jelly to the upper eyelid.
5. Reposition your client so that they are seated.
6. Work on only one eye at a time.
7. Using a lint free micro brush, carefully apply enough adhesive remover to cover the adhesive bonds on one eye.
8. Wait for 5 minutes for gel remover to work.
9. Gently manipulate the extensions off the natural eyelash using your tweezers, a micro wand or a cotton swab, being careful not to get gel remover on your clients face or in their eye.
10. Repeat the process until all extensions are removed.
11. Wipe away any excess adhesive remover using cotton swabs.
12. Cleanse any remaining adhesive remover using dampened cotton pads.
13. Discard soiled cotton pad and repeat until no adhesive remover remains and the eye area is completely clean.
14. Remove under eye barriers
15. Thoroughly rinse the eye area with distilled water or a saline solution formulated specifically for the eyes.
16. Repeat steps 6 through 15 on the other eye.
17. Brush and fan your client's eyelashes dry.
18. Have your client slowly open their eyes.
19. Follow with first aid if necessary.

Self Removal of Eyelashes

While it's not ever recommended that a client ever remove his or her own eyelash extensions, the need may arise due to an allergic or other reaction, and the inability to get a removal appointment booked right away. The client may also wish to remove their own lashes simply because they do not want to be exposed to the harsh chemical removers, or they don't want to pay for the removal service. If a client aims to remove their own eyelash extensions, they should proceed only with absolute caution, and knowledge that the process may take a number of hours, and that by removing the eyelash extensions themselves they risk prematurely pulling out their natural lashes. They should be informed that a prematurely plucked eyelash can take up to eight weeks to grow back, and repeated premature plucking of the eyelashes may lead to permanent eyelash loss.

Oils, including petroleum jelly and vegetable oils, are known to slowly break down the cyanoacrylate glue bonds. While removing an entire set of eyelash extensions using oil-based cleanser may take much longer than using a proper adhesive gel or cream-based remover, and using an oil to remove a single rogue lash, may prove to be impossible, it reduces exposure to chemicals, for your client (and you) in the long run.

A client who decides to remove their own eyelash extensions may attempt to do so by using a petroleum jelly, a pure coconut, olive or vegetable oil, or a heavy oil-based cleanser that will not hurt the eyes. With the eyes closed they may apply the oil to the eyelashes with a cotton pad. They may then gently rub the oil-soaked pad against their closed eyes and eyelashes, repeatedly, until the extensions slowly begin to fall off. This may be an extremely long process, with an average of just 3-4 extensions falling off every 20 minutes or so. I have attempted to remove my own extensions in this way, and I gave up long before the full set was removed!

If the client succeeds in self-removal, once all the lashes have been removed they should gently cleanse the oil from the eye area with warm, running water and a mild soap of their choice.

Chapter Summary Points

- With time, new natural eyelash growth will replace eyelashes with extensions attached.
- An eyelash extension artist should always have an eyelash adhesive remover on hand in case of emergency.
- Peeling an eyelash extension off a natural lash is safer than using an adhesive remover, when possible.
- Adhesive remover is extremely potent and should only be used sparingly.
- Every effort should be made, including having your client seated in an upright position, to ensure that adhesive remover does not touch the eyelid, or seep into the eye.
- If you suspect the adhesive remover got into the eye, follow with first aid for product contact with eye.
- While it is not recommended, a client may remove their own eyelashes if necessary, but they should be forewarned of the time it takes, and the potential to pull out, or harm, their own eyelashes.

14. Whoops! Fixing Things that have Gone Wrong

Applying eyelash extensions requires great dexterity, patience, and precision work. There are a few 'whoops!' moments that may occur along the way. This chapter is designed to help identify what's causing the problem and to help you find a solution.

Under Eye Pad Won't Stick

Some clients have extremely oily skin, strong lower lashes, and/or natural cavities around their eyes (especially at the inner corner) that make the under eye barrier pads quickly lose tack and come unstuck. Sometimes, this is just something you have to deal with by pressing the pads down frequently as you work. Other times, you may find there is a simple solution. Always make sure that your client has cleaned their eye area prior to their appointment. I keep an eyelash shampoo and eye cotton pads in my bathroom, so that clients can wash up properly before getting on the table. If the lashes are thick, and in cases where there is a natural cavity under the eye, tape the lashes down prior to applying the under eye pad. Be sure you are using a quality under eye pad that is not too thick. Thinner pads will stick better than thicker ones. And you may even purchase pads with, or choose to cut slits yourself in the bottom of the under eye pad to help it fit the contours of the client's face. The grey lines in the below diagram illustrate how you may cut the under eye pad to better fit the contours of your client's face.

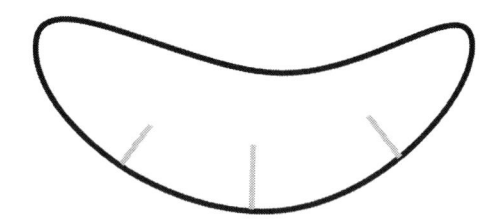

Lashes Stick Together During Application

No matter which pattern you use to apply eyelash extensions, having an extension stick to an extra natural lash, or to another extension along the way is inevitable. For this reason, the artist should do quick checks for lash separation throughout the application process. Checking the lashes after every 10-15 extensions applied should become habit. If you find anything stuck, gently peel the lashes apart using your tweezers. If you cannot peel the lashes apart, follow the instructions outlined for removing a rogue lash with adhesive remover. It's important not to leave the lashes stuck together as doing so will cause discomfort and will damage your client's natural lashes.

Sometimes, while inspecting lashes at the start of a fill appointment, you will find that the very tip of a lash is stuck to the base of an extension on another lash, and the shaft of the lash is angled in a sharp curve so that it forms something of a 'T' shape.

Extension applied to what apprears to be a single lash

With time you see a baby lash tip was adhered to the base of the extension

These baby lashes were at the very start of their anagen (growth) phase in close proximity to the mature lash that you applied the extension to. The lash you attached an extension to was in its telogen (resting) phase, and thus had completed growth. It's possible that the growing lash was so small at the time of your last appointment that you weren't able to see its tip growing into the base of the extension as you applied it. Now that it's grown out with it's tip stuck to the bottom of the old extension, it forms this T-junction with the lash it's stuck to. If there is enough space to slide both pairs of tweezers in, under the junction of the lashes, gently try to peel the lashes apart, without causing your client discomfort. If you aren't unable to do this you may either use your cosmetic scissors to cut only the misshaped lash being sure to apply a new extension to it immediately after, or you may follow the instructions outlined for removing a rogue lash with adhesive remover. Do not leave the lashes stuck together.

Lashes Keep Sticking to the Under Eye Pad
Sometimes, lashes get stuck to the under eye barrier. This may be caused by your client's closed-eye, eye movements (some people squint their eyes unintentionally, especially if they are talking or laughing), or by the angle of your client's head and face as they lay in a direction that causes the natural lashes to rest on the under eye pad. Straight, fine natural lashes

that are weighed down by extensions that are too heavy for them can also cause the lashes to stick to the under eye pad. While you're doing your periodic lash separation inspection you should be looking out for this and gently peeling any lashes off the bottom barrier as you find them. To help prevent it, make sure your client's head is angled in a position that causes their chin to slightly point up towards ceiling. This is achieved by keeping the bulk of any pillow under the neck and not under the head. You will also want to be sure that you are brushing the lashes frequently, before and as you are applying the extensions. Lashes should be brushed after every inspection. There is a taping technique outlined in the 'Tips & Tricks' section that may also help with this. And some eyelash extension artists will even use a heated eyelash curler to shape the lashes optimally prior to starting their application process. Remember that if you wish to use a heated curler, you should not use them on extensions that are already applied as heat may damage them and the client's natural lashes when extensions are applied, and that you will have to find a way to disinfect the curler between every client.

Lashes or Glue Gets Stuck To Upper Eyelid

If you drop a lash on your client's eyelid or face, you should be able to quickly but gently pick it up with the tweezers without causing any harm or discomfort. If a tiny speck of glue is left, you should advise your client of it. Let them know that the speck will disappear as their skin naturally sheds oils. You may also, and depending on the amount of glue dropped, wish to offer to remove it using an adhesive remover. If you must do this, remember the toxic nature of both the glue and the glue remover. You must follow with first aid for product contact with skin and/or eyes. Remember not to touch wet glue with cotton or wool products. The glue should be set with a mist of water, before you attempt to remove it. Once the glue and the glue remover has been wiped away, you must flush the area with distilled water or an eye rinse, for 15 minutes to ensure there is no reside left and to help prevent further reaction. See the 'First Aid' section, or your products Material Safety Data Sheet MSDS for more information on product contact with skin.

Old Extension Twists and/or Weighs the Lash Down

During the anagen phase the lashes grow rapidly. Remember in just 3-6 weeks a lash goes from non-existent to the telogen (transitional) phase. If you apply an extension to a lash that is at about half as long as it will naturally grow (or half way through it's anagen phase), in just 2 – 3 weeks it will be full length. If you apply a long extension to this growing lash, by the time your client returns for a fill appointment, the lash will now be full growth and the extension will be stuck closer to the end of the lash than the base. The weight distribution can cause the lash to twist, bend and even break the natural lash.

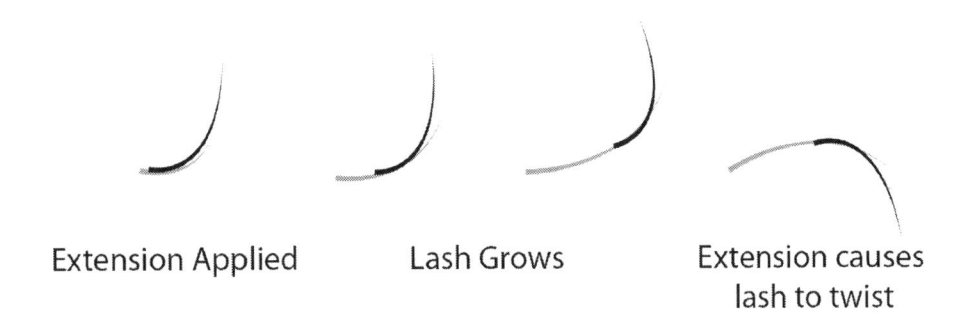

Extension Applied	Lash Grows	Extension causes lash to twist

Your client will most likely find this uncomfortable or annoying. For this reason, you should only apply short extensions to short lashes and long extensions to long lashes. It is inevitable though, that you sometimes break this rule in order to create a full, aesthetically pleasing set. If you can peel the old extension off without damaging the natural lash, do so. Alternatively, you may follow the instructions outlined for removing a rogue lash with adhesive remover.

Client Feels the Product is in Their Eye

If at any time the client feels there is product or product fumes in their eyes, fanning the lashes for a 20-30 seconds may help relieve the sensation. If this fails and/or if the sensation is perceived as an actual pain, you should flush the client's eye with distilled water or a saline solution formulated for use on the eyes. You can do this by having your client turn their face in the direction of the eye that needs flushing. Hold a paper towel under the side of the clients face, and use a squeeze bottle filled with distilled water or saline solution to flush the eye area. The client need not open their eye. Note, that this should not damage any of the extensions already applied. Once all pain or discomfort has been alleviated, pat dry the surrounding area. Brush the extensions using an eyelash wand while fanning away any remaining moisture. Re-prime the lashes and continue to apply the extensions.

There is a Gap in the Natural Lashes

A gap in the client's natural lash may be a natural occurrence, may be temporary or permanent traction alopecia, or some other condition. If the condition is not contraindicated, you'll wish to minimize its appearance. You can do this by doing what's referred to as bridging the gap. There are a couple of ways to do this. The first is by angling the extensions as you apply them to cover the gap. You may be able to close the gap by angling pre-built or hand-built fans towards the inside of the gap. If, for example, you are doing a Classic set of 0.15 lashes, you will want to create your bridge fans with 0.10 or 0.07 width extensions, depending on the strength of your client's natural lash and the size of the gap.

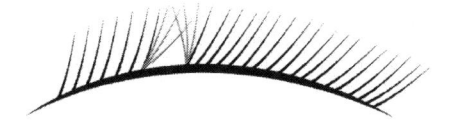

The term bridging the gap also sometimes applies to building an actual bridge over the gap. By placing a single lash, or even better, a small piece of your client's own natural hair, across the gap attaching it gently to strong natural lashes on either side of the gap, you effectively create a lash bridge. Make sure the lashes you are bridging are no longer growing and are in the catagen phase of the growth cycle. You may then apply very light, thinner extensions to the lash bridge itself, creating a fuller look of lashes.

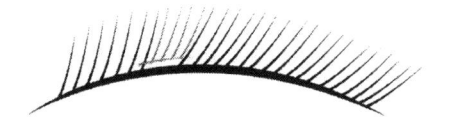

You can reinforce your bridge or give it more stability by placing two lashes, or pieces of hair, across the gap. Remember not to put too much weight on the natural lashes as you build fans to cover any gaps! Doing so may result in making the gap bigger by damaging the healthy natural lashes that are present!

Clients Eyes Are Twitchy While you Work

Twitchy eyes make it extremely hard to apply eyelash extensions and some clients are naturally twitchier than others. Twitching may be caused by your client talking, or rapid thoughts and even in clients who have fallen asleep. You will manage this depending on the cause. If the client is talking, politely ask them to stop, and explain why, so you don't come across as being rude.

If your client is deep in thought, you may find asking them to silently do breathing exercises may help. Explain to them that their eyes are twitching and ask them to attempt the 4-7-8 Breathing Exercise to slow it down. The instructions for 4-7-8 breathing are:

- Exhale completely through your mouth, making a whoosh sound.
- Close your mouth & inhale quietly through your nose to a mental count of 4.
- Hold your breath for a count of 7.
- Exhale through your mouth, making a whoosh sound, to a count of 8.
- This is one breath. Now, inhale again and repeat the cycle.

There is a link to more information on all the benefits of this exercise in the Resource section of this book. Alternatively, you may simply ask your client to take deep breaths and to concentrate their focus on their breathing.

If focusing on breathing and asking your client not to talk fails, you may find that putting a small piece of micropore tap, or an additional set of gel pads across the upper eyelids, stops the twitching. Placing a little weight on the top eyelid offers proprioceptive feedback to the nervous system that can help relax the eyelids while you work.

If your client has fallen asleep and the twitching is making it impossible for you to work, you have no choice but to wake them up. Remember, your client wants you to the best possible job you can do. They will help in whatever way they can to assist you with that!

Client Can't Open Eye as a Top Lash Stuck to the Bottom

Before you remove the under eye pad and have the client attempt to open their eyes, you should visually inspect to make sure that no upper lashes are stuck to the bottom. Using the wand, brush the eyelashes up to inspect the very bottom row. Sometimes, a lower lash will pop up from under the pad and an eyelash extension will be attached to it in error. This can be very uncomfortable for your client. The lash should be removed if caught before the client tries to open their eyes. If after your inspection, you still find that a lash or two is still stuck when your client attempts to open their eyes, gently try to manipulate it loose with your tweezers. Be extremely careful while your client is seated and you work with sharp tweezers near their eye. If you cannot separate the lash with your client seated, have them lie back down and try again. Sometimes, compressing the adhesive bond forcefully without applying any traction in the tweezers, can cause the bond to break and the extension to fall off. Use a small amount of adhesive remover only if necessary. Make sure it does not seep into their eyes. If any product has gotten onto the skin or into the eyes, you will have to follow this with first aid.

Eyelash Extensions Fall Out Prematurely

Having eyelashes extensions applied takes a long time and is costly. If the extensions fall out too soon, it can be extremely disappointing for your client, and for you, as all your hard work has gone to waste. Remember that it is natural for eyelashes to fall out at an average rate of 2-3 lashes per day. In the spring and summer time, we cycle through our lash growth and shed quicker. The natural life cycle of an eyelash means that in most circumstances, and for most people, the appropriate time to book fill appointments is every 2 to 3 weeks. If your client's lashes are falling out in large numbers prior to this, it's possible that you failed to thoroughly clean and prime the lashes at the start of your last appointment. Be sure not to skip this step! You may need to inspect the eyelashes to see if you failed to appropriately select or apply the extensions. If you chose extensions that are too heavy for the natural lash, it causes stress for the hair root, which may lead to the lash falling out. Apply lighter extensions. If you applied one extension to multiple natural lashes, or clumped natural lashes together with glue, this also causes the premature plucking and falling of the natural eyelashes. Be sure to isolate every single lash while applying extensions.

If you are certain that your procedure and your application technique are not the cause of the problem, it's possible that the client's natural anatomy, or their activities of daily living, are the cause. If the client is taking certain medications, has unusually oily skin, habitually touches or rubs their own lashes, or takes part in activities that cause them to sweat (including those hot flashes that come with menopause), frequent gentle cleansing of the eyelashes may help prevent the premature falling out. Remember that oils, both synthetic, and those that are naturally excreted by the skin, will slowly break down eyelash adhesive. Tears will also work to break down the adhesive bond, as will prolonged exposure to water or moisture.

Short duration exposure to water, like that of taking a shower, washing the face, or going for a quick swim, is not enough exposure to cause adhesive degradation. If your client is an avid swimmer, however, or a fitness enthusiast, or spends a great deal of time in any hot or humid area, or is simply just sweaty or oily (often due to medications or menopause), they may not be great candidates for eyelash extensions to begin with. It's important that they know these activities may lead to the premature falling out, or degeneration of the extensions, before they have the eyelash extensions applied.

It's not uncommon for one eye to lose eyelash extensions more frequently than the other. Sometimes, this is caused by the sleep position, and sometimes there is simply a natural discrepancy in the number of natural lashes, or the rate of eyelash growth cycles, or the amount of tearing or oil secretion that occurs in each eye. Asymmetry is normal and to be expected. As lash artists, we do our best to even out the appearance of asymmetrical lashes.

Eyelash Extensions Lose their Curl

Eyelash extensions may lose their curl because they were a low quality eyelash extension to begin with, or because your client spends a great deal of time in a hot and/or humid environment. Make sure your client is aware that this will occur in these conditions. They should not attempt to re-curl extensions with an eyelash curler. A manual eyelash curler may break the extension, the glue bond, or pull out the natural lashes and a heated eyelash extension curler will melt or burn the extensions and the natural lashes. Clients that must spend a great deal of time in a hot or moist environment may find that frequent brushing of the extensions helps prevent them from losing their curl. Otherwise, they will require more frequent fill appointments.

Eyelash Extensions are Itchy or Uncomfortable

Once the eyelash extensions have been applied, your client should not feel that they are there, beyond the acknowledgement that the extensions are longer and thicker than the natural eyelashes. Multiple lashes being adhered together may cause itchy or uncomfortable eyelash extensions. Remember that a faster growing lash will slowly pluck a slower growing lash, which will cause an itch sensation, pain or otherwise be uncomfortable! Lash isolation during application is important!

Eyelash extensions may also be itchy or uncomfortable due to bacteria growth. The space on the natural eyelash, between the eyelash extension and the eyelid is the perfect place for bacteria multiply. It is important that your client washes their face and eyelashes as normal, and does not hesitate to clean the eyelashes out of fear that the extensions will fall out.

If application technique and patient hygiene have been ruled out as the cause of itchy eyelashes, your client may be developing a sensitivity or allergy to the products used, or they may have a parasite infestation. If you suspect sensitivity, allergy or a lice infestation, remember that you do not have the necessary credentials to make a medical diagnosis. Do not diagnose your client. If you choose to do so, you may be wrong, and your suspicion may not only be offensive to your client, but may make you liable for the consequences of their actions based on what you tell them, whether or not you are right! Instead of offering a suggestion as to what is causing the itch, admit you do not know for certain, and tell your client that the best precaution for them to take is to remove the eyelash extensions immediately and to seek medical attention before another set is applied.

Generalized Red Eyes (Conjunctivitis) After Eyelash Extensions Applied

Conjunctivitis is a somewhat common immediate reaction to having eyelash extensions applied. Remember that we are using chemical irritants in close proximity to the eyeball. Even with the eyes closed, fumes will seep in. Sometimes clients will even open their eyes slightly, without realizing it. This is often the case if the client talks a lot during the application. Your client should not be in any pain at any time, even if red eyes occur. The eyes should not stay red for a prolonged period of time. If the eyes stay red for more than a day or two, your client should seek medical attention.

Using distilled water in a Nano mister or rinsing the extensions once fully applied to cure the adhesive, will help reduce the frequency of this happening.

Some eyelash extension artists will keep a soothing eye wash, or unopened over the counter eye drops on hand, in case their client requests them after having the eyelash extensions applied. Remember that you are not legally allowed to offer eye drops to your client, but you may give them unopened non-prescription eye cleansers if they ask for them. If the temporary conjunctivitis is a concern for your client, suggest they ask a chemist or pharmacist for the best solution.

Localized Red Eyes (Conjunctivitis) / Bruised Eyeball

If only the underside of the eyeball is red after the appointment, it's likely that the under eye pads, or tape, or both were either applied too close to the lash line, or they crept up into the closed eye during treatment. This often happens with chatty or twitchy clients. The localized conjunctivitis on the eyeball is referred to as an eye bruise.

The best way to avoid this is to be sure not to apply the lash pads too close to the lash line, and to ask your client not to chat or to move the eyes & face during the application. If eye-bruising doe occur, just like a regular skin bruise it may take a few days to disappear. Your client may wish to seek the care of a medical doctor.

Chapter Summary Points

- Applying eyelash extensions requires great dexterity, patience, and precision work. Mistakes happen along the way, and can be dealt with.
- There are various reasons why the under eye pad may not stick including your client's anatomy and physiology, or pad thickness. You can try multiple things to correct this including taping the eyelashes down first and placing the pad over top, using a thinner pad, or even cutting the pad.
- You should check frequently during the application for multiple lashes stuck together.
- It's often easy to prevent lashes from being stuck to the under eye pad by tilting the client's head slightly.
- Old, heavy extensions may weigh the natural lash down causing discomfort and damage to the hair follicle. These should be removed.
- Products in the eye should be followed up with first aid.
- By angling the extensions, or creating a lash bridge you can hide the appearance of a natural gap in the client's lashes.
- There are multiple reasons why extensions may fall out prematurely. Many of these reasons are due to application and many are due to the client's lash care. Troubleshooting is necessary for each client with poor retention.
- Heat and humidity are the main reasons why extensions lose their curl.
- If the extensions are itchy or uncomfortable it may be caused by poor application technique, or poor client hygiene. It may also be the onset of an allergy.
- A temporary bout of conjunctivitis after having eyelash extensions applied is normal for some people, especially those who open their eyes during the application. If it is prolonged, the client should seek medical attention.

- If eye bruising occurs you should make sure the eye pads are not placed too close to the eye, and ask your client not to chat during the appointment.

Definitions

Junction	a point where two or more things are joined
Twitching	give or cause to give a short, sudden jerking or convulsive movement
Proprioceptive	relating to stimuli that are produced and perceived within an organism, especially those connected with the position and movement of the body
Compressing	flatten by pressure; squeeze; press
Allergen	any substance that induces an allergy

15. Bad Eyelash Extensions / Good Eyelash Extensions

The work of an eyelash extension artist is extremely detailed, precision work that requires skill, patience, and practice. In an unregulated market, where many people are out to make a quick buck, there are a fair number of people offering this service, who lack one or all of the skills required to do a good job of it.

The below picture is a prime example of unskilled, sloppy work. In this photo that's widely shared over the Internet, you can see clumps of extensions stuck together, and multiple natural eyelashes adhered to various massive clumps. It also looks as though the eyelashes applied may have been too heavy for the natural lashes.

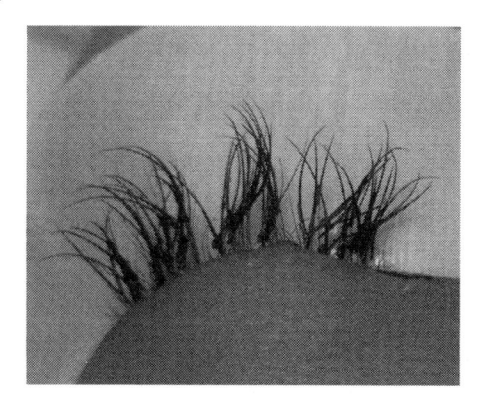

Notice how the heavier clumps of lashes have begun to curl to the side? Even a single overweight extension that is properly applied will begin to turn and will eventually break or pluck the natural lash. If left, this eyelash extension application would be extremely uncomfortable, would lead to traction alopecia, and possibly cause permanent damage of the eyelash follicles. The below photo, also shared on the Internet, shows what traction alopecia might look like, up close.

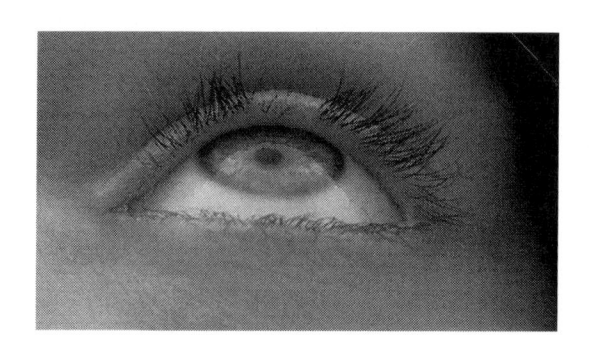

Lash isolation and separation is extremely important during the application process. When done correctly, the results are comfortable and visibly beautiful.

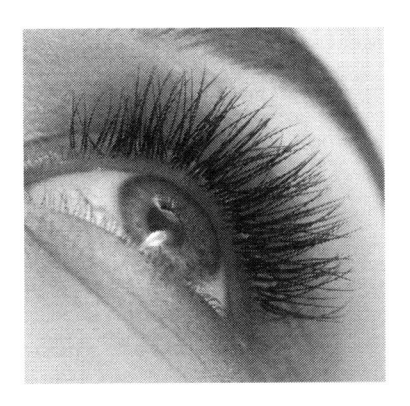

Good eyelash extensions that were applied with isolation skill and patience can turn bad with the inadequate care of your client. Some oils and other substances found in make-ups and creams, can cause the breakdown of the eyelash extension adhesive, which will partially liquefy and then re-solidify, attaching multiple eyelashes together in the process.

It is hard to assume with the following photo, whether or not these congealed clumps of lashes were caused by a poor initial application, or if this was caused by the improper care of the client. In this case, this new client advised the lash artist that she had never, ever washed her extensions. For this reason, you should not pass flash judgments on, or verbally speak poorly of someone else's work without full knowledge of the background.

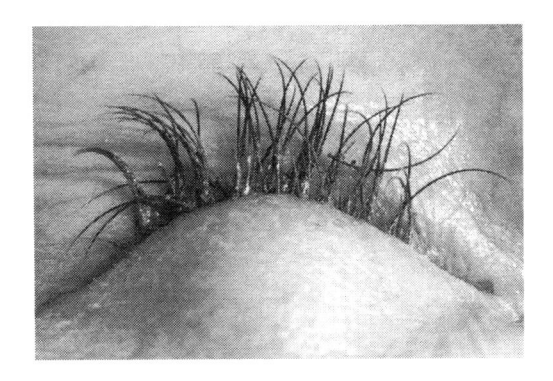

Should a client come to you with lashes that look like this, it is most professional to offer a full removal and thorough cleaning and if time permits, followed by a fresh application if the natural lashes are capable, and plenty of client education on the importance of proper cleansing and after care.

When extensions are done right, and are cared for by the client, they are comfortable, they look great, and will not damage the natural eyelash. The below photos show some of my favorite sets yet!

Classic:

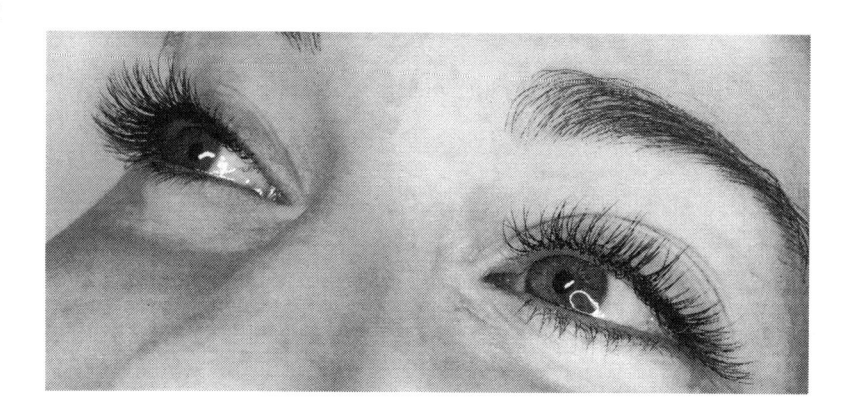

Russian Volume:

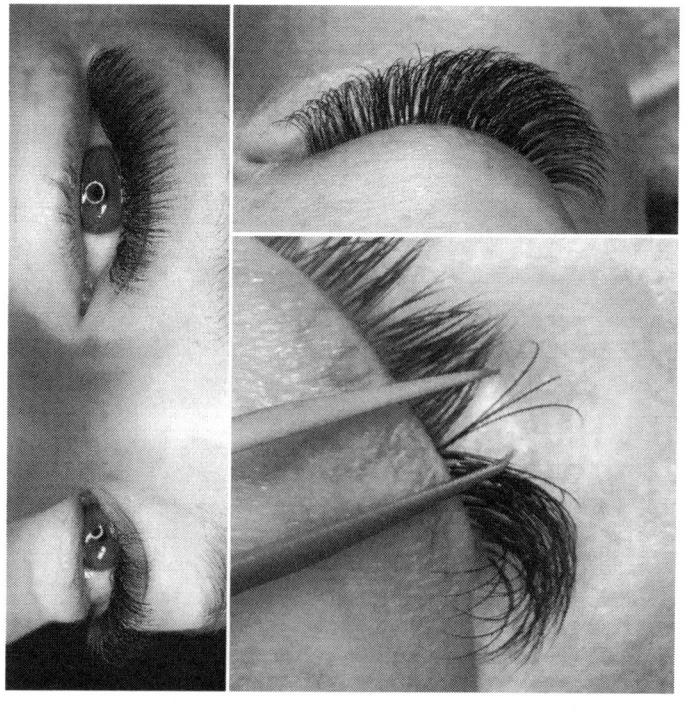

16. Closing Notes

You now have a great base of information related to the eyelash extension application industry. You have a good understanding of the anatomy and physiology of the eye and eyelashes. You can conceptualize the methods used to professionally apply and remove eyelash extensions. You understand the different abbreviations and terms used among eyelash extension artists, and the differences between a classic application, a volume application, and a Russian volume application. You know basic first aid procedures pertinent to the eyelash extension processes, and you're aware that you should have a proper certification in first aid while working with the public, in addition to this basic knowledge. You've been introduced to the legislative by-laws in British Columbia that are relevant to the personal service industry, and you're aware that if you are located elsewhere, you should look up and abide by the legislation of your area. What now?

Now, you must practice.

All the knowledge in the world won't perfect your application technique. Register in a proper hands-on, in-person course if you haven't already done so. Buy a practice mannequin and buy practice eyelashes, so you can practice until you're perfect. Practice basic classic application with 0.15mm width lashes, and become proficient at it before moving on to practice volume eyelash extensions. Practice with varying workstation set ups to determine what works best for you. And finally, once you've had some hands-on training beside a professional who can monitor your progress, practice on real people before you start charging for the service. Eyelash extension application is not easy. It requires precision work and a lot of patience. The work is extremely repetitive. Practice creating good habits from the beginning and you'll be an expert in no time.

Professional, eyelash extension materials can be purchased via the Clashes website at www.Clashes.ca. Our store is still growing, but aims to eventually carry everything you need to get started, including training mannequins and practice kits. Alternatively, you may find other online sources for materials. Just be careful that you are purchasing clean, quality materials and be prepared to wait extended times for delivery, and to pay potential import fees, especially when sourcing your products from distributors you are not familiar with, and from foreign countries. If you are lucky, there may even be an aesthetic store in your area that carries professional eyelash extension supplies.

I sincerely hope this book has been useful to you. I am wishing you all the best as you practice your new eyelash extension skills, become an eyelash extension artist, and grow your eyelash extension business! If you have any thoughts or feedback that you would like to share, I would love to hear from you. Please join us on our Facebook group at www.facebook.com/groups/ClashesExtensionForum/, get in touch via the www.Clashes.ca website or just email me directly at chrystal.ladouceur@gmail.com.

I so look forward to hearing from you!

Appendix

The documents that follow have been created for use in my own personal practice. I share them with you as templates so that you might modify them accordingly to suit your practice. Note that while my lawyer reviewed the liability waiver for its intended use in my practice, it does not serve as a legal document in yours. In order to ensure that your liability waiver is sound for your practice, you should have your own lawyer review the same.

Note that ready-to-print US Letter formatted PDF's of these forms can all be found on my website at www.Clashes.ca. Please feel free to download, edit and use as necessary.

Intake Form

First Name

Last Name

Email

Mobile Phone

Home Phone

Street Address

City

Province / Postal Code

Date of Birth

How did you hear about us?

Eyelash History

Is this your first time having eyelash extensions applied?
☐ Yes
☐ No

In the last 60 days, have you worn:
☐ Strip Lashes
☐ Flare Lashes
☐ Individual Lashes
☐ Other lashes
☐ None

Do you do any of the following to your natural eyelashes:
☐ Curl

☐ Tint
☐ Perm

These procedures cannot be done once eyelash extensions have been applied. If you wish to curl, tint or perm your natural eyelashes, please do so prior to extension application.

Are you having your eyelash extensions applied for:
☐ A special occasion
☐ Daily wear

Do you wear contact lenses?
☐ Yes – contact lenses must be removed prior to service
☐ No

Do you have or are you being treated for any eye illness or injury?
☐ Yes – please explain below
☐ No

Eye Illness or injury details:
_____

Please list any eye drops or eye medications that you use:
_____

Are you able to keep your eyes closed comfortably for more than 2 hours?
☐ Yes
☐ No

Please check any of the following that may apply to you:
☐ Lasik eye surgery
☐ Permanent eye make-up
☐ Blephoplasty (eye lift)
☐ Microdermabrasion
☐ Allergies – please describe here _____
☐ Childbirth within the last 120 days
☐ Major surgery within the last 120 days

- [ ] Alopecia**
- [ ] Hypersensitivity to cyanoacrylate, formaldehyde, any adhesives or glues
- [ ] Recent high fever or illness
- [ ] Regular exposure to swimming pool chemicals, bleach or dyes
- [ ] Drugs or medications that can cause temporary hair loss (Chemotheraputic drugs, Retinoids for acne treatment, Anticoagulants or Beta-adrenergic Blockers for blood pressure, etc)**

**Eyelash extensions cannot be bonded to skin. If you do not have natural eyelashes we cannot apply extensions. Alopecia sufferers or people taking medications that cause hair loss are not good candidates for this service.

Is there anything else you think we should know before you have your eyelash extensions applied?

_____

_____

Liability Waiver

Cancellation Policy

Your appointment time is reserved just for you. A late cancellation or missed visit leaves a hole in the eyelash extension artist's day that could have been filled by another client. As such, we require 24 hours notice for any cancellations or changes to your appointment. Clients that provide less than 24 hours notice or miss their appointment will be charged a cancellation fee.

☐ I Agree to the Cancellation Policy.

Waiver of Liability

I understand there are risks associated with having artificial eyelashes applied to and/or removed from my existing eyelashes, and that not withstanding the utmost of care in the application or removal of these products, there still exist risks associated with the procedure and product itself, which include, without limitation, eye irritation, eye pain, discomfort, and, in rare cases, blindness even when applied in the usual manner.

If I experience any irritation, redness, puffiness, itchiness, an allergic reaction or any other side effect of this procedure, I will contact a medical doctor immediately.

As part of this procedure, I understand that a certain amount of eyelash adhesive material will be used to attach the artificial eyelashes to my existing eyelashes. Even though the eyelash extension artist may apply or remove my eyelash extensions in the usual manner, I understand adhesive material may become dislodged during or after the procedure, which may irritate my eyes or require further follow-up care, at my own expense to prevent damage to my eyes. I also understand there is more than one technique for applying eyelash extensions to my eyelashes, and I will not attribute any liability to the eyelash extension artist as a result of this procedure or the use and care of these lashes.

As part of the removal procedure, I understand that a certain amount of chemical adhesive remover is applied to existing adhesives and a reaction occurs to dissolve the adhesive that results in the thinning of the remover.

Even though the eyelash extension artist may apply or remove my eyelash extensions in the usual manner, I understand the liquid remover may seep into my eyes, which may irritate my eyes or require further follow-up care, at my own expense to prevent damage to my eyes.

I also agree to defend, indemnify and hold harmless the eyelash extension artist from any and all claims, actions, expenses, damages and liabilities, including reasonable attorneys' fees which might be asserted against her as a result of my having this procedure performed, or my purchase of these eyelash extension products from her.
☐ I Agree to this Waiver of Liability.

Permissions to Use Photographs

I hereby grant the eyelash extension artist the full right to take, publish and reproduce photographs of me, my face, my eyes and/or eyelashes, both before and after this procedure, for any advertising, education, or other purposes whatsoever, including the right to retouch these photographs as deemed necessary by the eyelash extension artist. I further expressly assign any copyright in these photographs to the eyelash extension artist. I also grant my consent for the eyelash extension artist to use my image and likeness as contained in these photographs for any advertising or other purposes
☐ I Agree.

Care and Maintenance

I agree to follow the care and maintenance instructions provided by the eyelash extension artist for the use and care of my eyelash extensions, and that if any follow up care is required due to my own mistake or negligence, or failure to follow these instructions, this will be at my own expense and risk. I understand that if I do any of the following, it may result in damage to my eyelash extensions or may cause my lashes to fall off prematurely. Knowing this I agree to follow these tips for best results:
*I will avoid oil based eye products, as these will loosen the bond of my eyelash extensions.
*If I experience any itching or irritation, I agree to contact a medical doctor immediately and the eyelash extension artist to have the eyelash extensions removed.

*I agree to avoid using waterproof mascara and to not use an eyelash curler, perm, or tint my eyelash extensions.
*I agree to not pick, pull or rub my eyelash extensions.
*I understand that I should not attempt to remove my lash extensions on my own or with any product, but that the procedure requires that my eyelash extensions be professionally removed.
I understand that if I pick, pull on, or rub my eyelash extensions it may result in the premature temporary and permanent loss of my artificial and natural eyelashes.
☐ I Agree to the Care and Maintenance Terms.

No Known Medical Conditions / Informed Consent

I have read and completed the Eyelash Extension Intake Form in its entirety and in truth. I acknowledge that I have been advised of the potential harmful or negative side effects (such as the premature shedding of my eyelash) that the lash extension procedure or removal may cause to those who have specific medical or skin conditions. I understand that the adhesives and adhesive remover are a skin, eye and mucus membrane irritant and that in rare cases persons may be allergic or have hypersensitivity to synthetics, cyanoacrylate or formaldehyde, which in small amount may be present in the adhesive. I understand that the procedure requires that I lay still for up to 2 hours or longer with my eyes shut, and that if I wear contacts, I must remove my contact lenses for the duration of the lash extension application or removal. I further state that I have no known medical condition that might be aggravated by the procedure or any medical condition that would prevent me from complying with or heeding to the eyelash extension artist's instructions or these warnings.
☐ I Agree.

Spot Test

I understand, that should I have any concerns about any possible reaction to chemicals and products used, I may arrange at my own discretion to book an advance spot test where 2 to 3 individual lashes will be applied 24-48 hours prior to the time in which I'm scheduled for my initial full set. I further agree, that this shall be my own responsibility and at my sole

discretion, and have absolutely no bearing on the contents or signing of this agreement or any clauses contained therein.
☐ I Agree.

Full Name: _____

Signature: _____

Date: _____

Client Record – Lash History

Client Name

_____

Date of Appointment

_____

Lash Brand / Type   Lash Lengths Used

_____   _____

Curl(s)   Lash Widths

_____   _____

Appointment & Style Notes

_____

_____

_____

~*~

Date of Appointment

_____

Lash Brand / Type   Lash Lengths Used

_____   _____

Curl(s)   Lash Widths

_____   _____

Appointment & Style Notes

_____

_____

_____

Immediately Post Application
- Wash face as usual.
- For maximal bonding avoid touching the lashes for 24-hours.
- Do not swim, bath, steam or spend any prolonged amount of time with the eyelashes wet.
    - If these are your regular activities and they will break down the eyelash adhesive and cause premature eyelash loss. Fills may need to be applied more frequently

Extended Care
- Be gentle with your eyelashes. Do not pull on the eyelids or rub the eyes.
- Do not use oil-based products on or around the eyelashes.
- Clean your eyelashes regularly using a mild oil-free soap and water. Gently pat dry. Do not rub.
- If mascara is required, use water-soluble mascara only.
- Use powdered, liquid or gel eyeliners. Pencils (unless specially formulated for eyelash extensions) tend to leave an oily residue, which could loosen the bond.
- Do not use eyelash curlers.
- Do not tint or perm the eyelash extensions – any tinting must be done before extensions are applied.
- Avoid blasts of direct heat as this can cause the lash extensions to lose shape and/or burn the lashes. (Step aside when opening the oven/BBQ or if you are a smoker, turn the cigarette away from yours eyes when lighting)
- Never pull off the eyelash extensions as this will pull out your natural eyelashes.
- Do not remove the eyelash extensions on your own. If you need the extensions removed set up an appointment with a professional.

References & Further Learning Materials

Clashes Main Website	www.Clashes.ca
Clashes Understanding Allergies	http://clashes.ca/understanding-eyelash-extension-allergies/
Clashes Online Shop	www.peninsulashes.com
Dumont Tweezers	http://dumonttweezers.com/
Fine Science Tools	http://www.finescience.ca/
Eyelash Extension Artist Facebook Group	www.facebook.com/groups/ClashesExtensionForum/
Guidelines for Personal Service Establishments (PSEs)	http://www2.gov.bc.ca/gov/content/health/keeping-bc-healthy-safe/pses-mpes#pse
Direct link to Guidelines for PSEs	http://www2.gov.bc.ca/assets/gov/health/keeping-bc-healthy-safe/pses/pse-guidelines.pdf
Seasonality of Hair Shedding Study	https://www.ncbi.nlm.nih.gov/pubmed/19407435
4-7-8 Breathing	http://aspecthealth.ca/4-7-8-breathing/
Difference between isopropyl and rubbing alcohol	http://www.differencebetween.com/difference-between-isopropyl-and-vs-rubbing-alcohol/
Gray's Anatomy – Anatomy of the Human Body	http://www.bartleby.com/107/
Clorox Disinfecting Bleach Chemical Information link	http://www.cloroxprofessional.ca/products/ultra-clorox-disinfecting-bleach/
How Super Glue is Made	http://www.madehow.com/Volume-1/Super-Glue.html
Histotoxicity of Cyanoacrylate Tissue Adhesive in the Rat	https://www.ncbi.nlm.nih.gov/pmc/articles/PMC1476793/

Made in the USA
San Bernardino, CA
01 October 2017